CHAPTER 1

INTRODUCTION

> Besides natural disasters and naturally occurring novel infectious diseases, nothing potentially threatens the health and stability of nations and health systems as much as the devastating threat and unfathomability of bioterrorism.
> — Gregory A. Poland et al., "The Social, Political, Ethical, and Economic Aspects of Biodefense Vaccines"

Background

Anthrax is considered one of the most likely biological warfare agents because of the ability of anthrax spores to be transmitted by the respiratory route, the high mortality of inhalation anthrax, and the dramatic stability of anthrax spores compared with other potential biological warfare agents.[1] Anthrax has been the focus of offensive and defensive biological warfare research programs in various nations for approximately 60 years.[2] During World War I, the Germans deliberately exposed horses and cattle to anthrax before the animals were shipped to France.[3] In World War II, Japan researched the effects of aerosolized anthrax on prisoners of war.[4] The United Sates maintained a research and development program for offensive biological agents between 1943 and

---

[1] Advisory Committee on Immunization Practices, "Use of Anthrax Vaccine in the United States," *MMWR Recommendations and Reports* 49 (15 December 2000): 2.

[2] Ibid.

[3] Robert G. Darling and Jon B. Woods, ed., *USAMRIID's Medical Management of Biological Casualties Handbook*, 5th ed. (Frederick, MD: U.S. Army Medical Research Institute Of Infectious Diseases, 1994), 2.

[4] Ibid.

1969.[5] The United States weaponized anthrax spores in the 1950s and 1960s.[6] Following the halt of offensive biological and toxin weapon research in 1969, the US Army Medical Research Institute of Infectious Diseases (USAMRIID) has maintained a biological defense program to include ongoing study of anthrax.[7]

Anthrax vaccines for animal use were developed initially in the 19th century.[8] Human anthrax vaccines were developed in the 1950s, and were tested on human subjects in the 1960s.[9] The Anthrax Vaccine Adsorbed (AVA) was licensed for human use in the United States in 1970.[10] Following licensure, patients with occupational risk for anthrax exposure, such as veterinarians, research scientists, and textile mill workers, commonly received the anthrax vaccine.[11] The US Food and Drug Association (FDA) and the vaccine manufacturer report that approximately 68,000 doses of human anthrax vaccine were dispensed between 1974 and 1989.[12] Approximately 1,500 Department of Defense

---

[5]Ibid., 3.

[6]Ibid., 18.

[7]Ibid., 3.

[8]Committee to Assess the Safety and Efficacy of the Anthrax Vaccine, Medical Follow-Up Agency, *The Anthrax Vaccine: Is It Safe? Does It Work?* (Washington, DC: National Academies Press, 2002), 40.

[9]Peter C. B. Turnbull, ―Anthrax Vaccines: Past, Present, and Future,‖ *Vaccine* 9 (1991): 533.

[10]Committee to Assess the Safety and Efficacy of the Anthrax Vaccine and Medical Follow-Up Agency, 40.

[11]Ibid.

[12]Military Vaccine (MILVAX) Agency, Office of the Army Surgeon General, ―Anthrax Vaccine Immunization Program (AVIP) Questions and Answers,‖

(DoD) laboratory workers have utilized the anthrax vaccine since FDA approval in 1970.[13]

In 1979, an apparent accidental release of anthrax spores from a military microbiology facility in Sverdlovsk, Russia, resulted in 79 reported cases of inhalational anthrax and 68 deaths.[14] In the 1980s and 1990s, several nations developed and enhanced their biological weapons programs. Growing concern about the use of anthrax as a biological weapon led to vaccination of limited numbers of United States military personnel in the early 1990s.[15] Approximately 150,000 US service members received the licensed anthrax vaccine during the first Gulf War.[16] In August 1991, Iraqi government representatives disclosed to the United Nations Special Commission Team investigating Iraq's bioweapons capabilities that Iraq had conducted research into the offensive use of anthrax.[17] In 1995, United Nations inspectors gained additional information on Iraq's offensive bioweapons program: ―In December 1990, the Iraqis filled 100 R400 bombs with botulinum toxin, 50 with anthrax, and 16 with aflatoxin. In addition, 13 Al Hussein

---

http://www.anthrax.osd.mil/documents/Anthrax_QA.pdf (accessed 23 November 2010), 6.

[13]Ibid.

[14]Committee to Assess the Safety and Efficacy of the Anthrax Vaccine and Medical Follow-Up Agency, 42.

[15]Ibid., 40.

[16]Ibid., 3.

[17]Darling and Woods, 4.

(SCUD) warheads were filled with botulinum toxin, 10 with anthrax, and 2 with aflatoxin."[18]

In 1992, Ken Alibek, a senior Russian bioweapons program manager defected to the United States. Mr. Alibek disclosed details of a robust Soviet bioweapons program with the capacity to produce large quantities of various agents.[19] In the 1990s, following the fall of the Soviet Union, growing concern existed in the United States about the transfer of bioweapons knowledge and capabilities to hostile states.[20] Responding to this threat, in December 1997, Secretary of Defense William Cohen announced a plan to universally vaccinate all United States service members with the anthrax vaccine.[21] In March 1998, the Anthrax Vaccine Immunization Program (AVIP) began.[22] In July 1999, Secretary of the Air Force F. Whitten Peters told the Senate Armed Services Committee that ―[Anthrax] has been weaponized and we know it is deployed in about 10 countries around the world." [23] Alarmingly, in the fall of 2001, anthrax was used successfully for

---

[18]Ibid.

[19]Ibid., 5.

[20]Ibid.

[21]Committee to Assess the Safety and Efficacy of the Anthrax Vaccine and Medical Follow-Up Agency, 33.

[22]Ibid.

[23]Jim Davis and Anna Johnson-Winegar, ―The Anthrax Terror DOD's Number-One Biological Threat," *Aerospace Power Journal* (Winter 2000): 24.

bioterrorism within the United States.[24] Letters containing anthrax spores were sent to members of Congress and the media, sickening 17 people, and killing five.[25]

Safety, efficacy, policy, and legal concerns surrounded the AVIP in the late 1990s and early to mid-2000s. Impaired production capacity, fears regarding adverse events associated with the vaccine, patient refusals, licensing irregularities, changing policies, and legal injunctions challenged vaccine delivery. By 2001, more than 400 service members who refused anthrax vaccinations had left the military either voluntarily or involuntarily.[26] Further, a 2000 General Accounting Office (GAO) survey of Air National Guard and Air Force Reserve pilots and aircrew personnel found that respondents cited the mandatory anthrax immunization as a primary reason for leaving the military.[27]

Significant public concern regarding the vaccine and administration policies prompted Congress to direct the DoD to support an independent examination of the AVA by the National Academy of Sciences' Institute of Medicine in 2000.[28] In 2005, the FDA reviewed the AVA and found it to be ―safe and effective for its labeled indication to

---

[24]Centers for Disease Control and Prevention, ―Update: Investigation of Bioterrorism-Related Anthrax and Interim Guidelines for Clinical Evaluation of Persons with Possible Anthrax," *Morbidity and Mortality Weekly Report* 50, no. 43 (2 November 2001): 941.

[25]Federal Bureau of Investigation, ―Amerithrax Investigation," http://www.fbi.gov/anthrax/amerithraxlinks.htm (accessed 15 September 2010).

[26]Committee to Assess the Safety and Efficacy of the Anthrax Vaccine and Medical Follow-Up Agency, 85.

[27]United States General Accounting Office, GAO-01-92T, *Anthrax Vaccine Preliminary Results of GAO's Survey of Guard/Reserve Pilots and Aircrew Members* (Washington, DC: Government Printing Office, 11 October 2000), 2.

[28]Committee to Assess the Safety and Efficacy of the Anthrax Vaccine and Medical Follow-Up Agency, 34.

protect individuals at high risk for anthrax disease."[29] Since 2007, the AVA has been administered to all service members not medically or administratively exempt deploying to high-threat areas.

Marked changes in patient education, vaccine tracking, vaccine risk and benefit communication, AVA schedule, and AVA delivery have occurred within the past three years. Despite these changes, vocal opponents of the AVIP exist. Opponents question the disease threat, vaccine safety and efficacy, vaccine indications, and adverse vaccine reactions. Historical fears surrounding the AVA have included a possible association with Gulf War Syndrome, association with severe adverse events, and vaccine adjuvant contents.

Problem Statement

The AVA is intended to protect against a feared, but invisible and intangible threat. The AVIP was has a convoluted and controversial history, and has undergone multiple changes. Recent studies have added additional evidence-based information about AVA safety and efficacy to the scientific literature. The DoD regularly assesses risks and benefits of all force protection measures. The risks and benefits of the AVIP for individual service members and as a force protection strategy require ongoing assessment.

---

[29]Department of Health And Human Services, Food and Drug Administration, ―Biological Products; Bacterial Vaccines and Toxoids; Implementation of Efficacy Review; Anthrax Vaccine Adsorbed; Final Rule and Final Order," *Federal Register* 70, no. 242 (19 December 2005), 75180-98, http://www.fda.gov/ohrms/dockets/ 98fr/05-24223.pdf (accessed 15 September 2010).

Research Question

Based on available evidence-based literature, what are the current known risks and benefits of the AVIP?

Thesis Statement

This study will identify and address current risks and benefits associated with the AVIP. To fully understand the AVIP, the disease, available treatments, vaccine safety and efficacy, and the vaccine's role in force protection are reviewed. The historical use and current use of the vaccine are detailed. Prior controversies surrounding the vaccine are addressed. The risks associated with the anthrax vaccine to include financial costs, opportunity costs, risk of adverse reactions for service members, and risks for the force will be compared with benefits for service members and benefits for the force.

Scope of Research

Further described in Chapter 3, Methodology, this study is qualitative and descriptive in nature. The known financial costs, opportunity costs, risk(s) for individuals, risk(s) for force health protection, financial benefit(s) for individuals, financial benefit(s) for force health protection, health benefit(s) for individuals, and health benefit(s) for force health protection associated with the AVIP are detailed and compared.

Limitations

The current study does not address force protection strategies related to alternate vaccines, bioterrorism unrelated to anthrax, or suspected adverse reactions related to other vaccines. The current study specifically queries risks and benefits of the AVIP for service members who receive the vaccine secondary to deployment to high-threat areas. The current study does not address the risk and benefit matrix for service members that have a primary occupational indication for anthrax vaccination, such as veterinarians, laboratory personnel, and other personnel with regular occupational exposure to anthrax.

Organization of Thesis

Chapter 2 reviews scholarly literature and previous research relevant to the AVA and AVIP. Chapter 2 includes a clinical review of anthrax disease, an overview of anthrax disease and its epidemiology, human manifestations of anthrax disease, anthrax prevention strategies, anthrax mitigation strategies, relevance of anthrax as a bioterrorism threat, overview of the anthrax vaccine, anthrax vaccine efficacy, anthrax vaccine safety, history of AVIP policy, current AVIP policy, and divergent opinions regarding AVIP policy. Chapter 3 describes the research methodology in detail. This description includes a model for comparison of risks and benefits associated with AVIP. Chapter 4 provides the findings of the analysis. Based on the findings, chapter 5 provides recommendations for consideration regarding future AVIP strategies.

Summary

This chapter introduced a research problem regarding the AVIP. This chapter identified the research question, scope, limitations, and the organization of this thesis paper. Chapter 2 will review the scholarly literature and previous research related to the AVIP.

CHAPTER 2

LITERATURE REVIEW

Anthrax is one of the great infectious diseases of antiquity.
— Theodore J. Cieslak and Edward M. Eitzen, Jr.,
─Clinical and Epidemiologic Principles of Anthra"

Introduction

This purpose of this chapter is to provide the clinical, scientific, and historical framework necessary to understand the development of, and historical controversies surrounding the current AVIP. In order to provide a thorough background, this chapter is organized into 12 sections. These sections provide background, support the thesis research question, and support the thesis methodology. The sections are (1) a clinical overview of anthrax disease; (2) an overview of anthrax disease and its epidemiology; (3) human manifestations of anthrax disease; (4) anthrax prevention strategies; (5) anthrax mitigation strategies; (6) relevance of anthrax as a bioterrorism threat; (7) overview of the anthrax vaccine; (8) anthrax vaccine efficacy; (9) anthrax vaccine safety; (10) history of AVIP policy; (11) current AVIP policy; and (12) divergent opinions regarding AVIP policy.

Anthrax Disease

Anthrax is an infectious zoonotic disease caused by the resilient, spore-forming bacterium *Bacillus anthracis* (*B. anthracis*).[30] Anthrax is common throughout the world

---

[30]Emergent BioSolutions, ─BioThrax® (Anthrax Vaccine Adsorbed)," http://www.fda.gov/downloads/BiologicsBloodVaccines/BloodBloodProducts/Approved Products/LicensedProductsBLAs/UCM074923.pdf (accessed 2 September 2010).

in wild and domestic vertebrate herbivores to include cattle, sheep, and goats.[31] Human disease occurs with exposure to infected animals, exposure to tissue from infected animals, and direct exposure to *B. anthracis*.[32]

Disease Background and Epidemiology

Human anthrax outbreaks have occurred throughout recorded history.[33] The Biblical fifth and sixth plagues in the book of Exodus may have been bovine and human anthrax.[34] Anthrax swept through Europe in the 1600s as the ―Black Bane,‖ causing both animal and human deaths.[35] Robert Koch, a German physician and bacteriologist, isolated the anthrax bacterium in 1876.[36] In 1881, Louis Pasteur announced an attenuated, live veterinary anthrax vaccine.[37]

B. anthracis is a variable part of normal soil flora. When local multiplication occurs and the number of organisms in the soil increase, the risk of infection in grazing animals increases. Conditions that favor *B. anthracis* growth include increasing soil pH, a

---

[31]Centers for Disease Control and Prevention, National Center for Zoonotic, Vector-Borne, and Enteric Diseases, ―Anthrax,‖ http://www.cdc.gov/nczved/ divisions/dfbmd/diseases/anthrax/#how_common (accessed 10 September 2010).

[32]Advisory Committee on Immunization Practices, ―Use of Anthrax Vaccine in the United States,‖ 1.

[33]Theodore J. Cieslak and Edward M. Eitzen Jr., ―Clinical and Epidemiologic Principles of Anthrax,‖ *Emerging Infectious Diseases* 5, no. 4 (July-August 1999): 552.

[34]Ibid.

[35]Ibid.

[36]Ibid.

[37]Kendall A. Smith, ―Wanted, an Anthrax Vaccine: Dead or Alive?‖ *Medical Immunology* 4, no. 5 (18 April 2005): 3, http://www.medimmunol.com/content/ pdf/1476-9433-4-5.pdf (accessed 17 October 2010).

rich concentration of organic matter, and changes in the soil microenvironment secondary to increased rainfall or drought.[38] *B. anthracis* forms spores when environmental conditions are not conducive to growth of bacilli.[39] Spore forms are resistant to heat, cold, pH, desiccation, chemicals, and irradiation.[40] Spore forms are the predominant environmental phase.[41] When a host ingests spores, the spores germinate and subsequently produce vegetative forms that multiply and eventually kill the host.[42] Bacilli then spread into the environment, subsequently sporulate, and are taken up by another animal.[43]

Biological warfare experiments on the island of Gruinard, off the western coast of Scotland, demonstrate the durability of anthrax spores. Gruinard was the site of biological warfare experiments in 1942 and 1943.[44] Approximately 4.0×10^{14} spores were explosively dispersed onto Gruinard.[45] Annual tests for more than 20 years demonstrated

---

[38]F. Marc LaForce, ―Anthrax,‖ *Clinical Infectious Diseases*, 19 (December 1994): 1010.

[39]P. C. B. Turnbull, ―Guidelines for the Surveillance and Control of Anthrax in Human and Animals. 3rd ed.,‖ *World Health Organization Emerging and other Communicable Diseases, Surveillance and Control WHO/EMC/ZDI/98.6*: 2, http://www.who.int/csr/resources/publications/anthrax/whoemczdi986text.pdf (accessed 18 October 2010).

[40]Ibid., 1.

[41]Ibid.

[42]Ibid.

[43]Ibid.

[44]LaForce, 1010.

[45]Ibid.

continued presence of anthrax spores.[46] Following sampling in 1986, 200 tons of formaldehyde diluted in 2000 tons of seawater and topsoil removal was used to disinfect contaminated areas.[47] In 1987, sampling studies did not demonstrate anthrax spores, and the island returned to agricultural use.[48]

Human anthrax most commonly results from direct or indirect contact with infected animals. World Health Organization (WHO) 1997 surveillance data characterize anthrax as enzootic in Africa, Asia, countries in Europe, areas of the American continent, and parts of Australia.[49] Anthrax infections occur sporadically within many additional countries.[50] More than 6,000 human anthrax cases occurred in Zimbabwe during 1979-1980.[51] Twenty five people developed anthrax in Paraguay in 1987 following the slaughter of an infected cow.[52] In October 2010, an anthrax outbreak in Bangladesh spread throughout 12 districts, infected more than 600 people with cutaneous anthrax, and killed cattle.[53]

---

[46]Ibid.

[47]Ibid.; BBC News, ―Britain's ‗Anthrax Island‗,‖ 25 July 2001, http://news.bbc.co.uk/1/hi/scotland/1457035.stm (accessed 2 December 2010).

[48]LaForce, 1010.

[49]Turnbull, ―Guidelines for the Surveillance and Control of Anthrax in Human and Animals,‖ 1.

[50]Ibid.

[51]Cieslak and Eitzen, 552.

[52]Ibid.

[53]James Melik and Anbarasan Ethirajan, ―Anthrax Outbreak Hits Bangladesh Leather and Meat Sectors,‖ *BBC News*, 13 October 2010, http://www.bbc.co.uk/news/business-11451570 (accessed 17 October 2010).

In the United States, anthrax infections have been infrequent since the 1970s.[54] The United States Centers for Disease Control and Prevention (CDC) investigated 49 cases of anthrax between 1950 and 2001.[55] Of these 49 investigations, 84 percent involved human or animal infections, two were evaluations of decontamination of anthrax–contaminated textile mills, and one was an investigation of a bioterrorism threat involving anthrax in 1998.[56] In the other five investigations, *B. anthracis* was not found to be the causative organism, despite initial suspicion.[57]

Human Manifestations of Disease

Symptoms of anthrax vary depending on the route of infection.[58] Approximately 95 percent of anthrax infections are cutaneous, associated with handling contaminated products from infected animals.[59] Cutaneous disease causes primarily local injury with corresponding local lymphatic response. Approximately 20 percent of untreated cutaneous anthrax cases result in mortality.[60] With appropriate antimicrobial therapy,

---

[54]Daniel B. Jernigan et al., "Investigation of Bioterrorism-Related Anthrax, United States, 2001: Epidemiologic Findings," *Emerging Infectious Diseases* 8, no. 10 (2002): 1019.

[55]Michael Bales et al., "Epidemiologic Response to Anthrax Outbreaks: Field Investigations, 1950-2001," *Emerging Infectious Diseases* 8, no. 9 (2002): 1163.

[56]Ibid., 1164.

[57]Ibid.

[58]Centers for Disease Control and Prevention, "Anthrax."

[59]Ibid.

[60]Ibid.

death from cutaneous anthrax is rare.[61] Gastrointestinal anthrax is associated with

consumption of contaminated meat.[62] Symptoms include abdominal pain, vomiting of

blood, diarrhea, difficulty swallowing, and marked swelling of the lymphatic tissue of the

throat and neck.[63] Morbidity results in 25 percent to 60 percent of cases of

gastrointestinal anthrax.[64] Inhalational anthrax initially resembles a non-specific upper

respiratory infection. Symptoms typically progress over several days to severe respiratory

distress and shock. Despite modern, aggressive antibiotic therapy and supportive care, 45

percent of inhalation anthrax cases from the 2001 bioterrorist attacks within the United

States were fatal.[65]

The virulence of anthrax strains is related to the presence of a three component

protein exotoxin composed of edema factor (EF), lethal factor (LF), and protective

antigen (PA).[66] EF causes edema.[67] LF causes cell death through an unknown

mechanism.[68] However, neither can produce these deleterious effects without the

presence of PA.[69] PA initially binds to cell surface receptors, a small piece of PA is

---

[61]Ibid.

[62]Ibid.

[63]Ibid.

[64]Ibid.

[65]Ibid.

[66]LaForce, 1009.

[67]Ibid.

[68]Ibid.

[69]Ibid.

cleaved, and then a binding site for either LF or EF becomes available.[70] Once associated with the PA, EF or LF can move inside the cell cytosol, causing damage to the cell and to the host.[71]

Disease Prevention Strategies

The anthrax vaccine is the only known effective pre-exposure prevention measure against anthrax.[72] Post-exposure disease prevention measures include oral antibiotics and vaccination. The CDC currently recommends 60 days of oral antibiotics and a three-dose regimen of anthrax vaccine for post-exposure prophylaxis in the event of exposure to *B. anthracis.*[73] The Advisory Committee on Immunization Practices (ACIP) and the Johns Hopkins Working Group on Civilian Biodefense, concur that based on available data, the best means for prevention of inhalation anthrax following exposure is a lengthy antibiotic course in concert with anthrax vaccination.[74] An Institute of Medicine Report (IOM) on anthrax vaccine safety and efficacy also concluded that based on animal studies, post-exposure prophylaxis should include anthrax vaccine administered in concert with antibiotics.[75]

---

[70]Ibid., 1010.

[71]Ibid.

[72]Centers for Disease Control and Prevention, Emergency Preparedness and Response, ─Anthrax Q and A: Preventive Therapy," http://www.bt.cdc.gov/agent/ anthrax/faq/preventive.asp (accessed 19 October 2010).

[73]Ibid.

[74]Ibid.

[75]Ibid.

Disease Mitigation Strategies

In patients with anthrax disease, the primary therapy is a tailored antibiotic regimen. Bacterial susceptibility testing and patient clinical status determine antibiotic selections.[76] In the late 1800s and early 1900s animal and human antisera were used for the treatment of anthrax infections.[77] The 1943 US Army medical supply catalog included human anthrax antiserum.[78] Although no controlled human studies demonstrate the efficacy of anthrax antiserum, experimental evidence indicates that antiserum given before or immediately after spore challenge prevents anthrax disease in guinea pigs, rhesus monkeys, and rats.[79] Anthrax immunoglobulin was used in successful treatment of a 2006 case of inhalational anthrax in the United States.[80] The US Strategic National Stockpile does include therapeutic courses of human polyclonal anthrax immunoglobulin manufactured from fractionated plasma of volunteers who previously had received four or more doses of AVA.[81]

---

[76]John D. Grabenstein, "Countering Anthrax: Vaccines and Immunoglobulins," *Clinical Infectious Diseases* 45 (15 December 2007): 133.

[77]Ibid.

[78]Ibid.

[79]Ibid.

[80]Ibid., 134.

[81]Ibid., 133.

Anthrax as a Bioterrorism Threat

―From a biological warfare perspective, it [anthrax] is the poor-man's/poor country's weapon of mass destruction."[82] Anthrax infection is highly lethal, stable, and readily available in the environment.[83] The US Congress Office of Technology Assessment estimated that 220 pounds of anthrax delivered from an aircraft in Washington, DC, would result in up to three million casualties pending ideal weather conditions.[84] As compared to other known bioweapons, a small amount of anthrax has tremendous destructive potential. Oak Ridge National Laboratories demonstrated that 1,763 pounds of sarin nerve gas, 0.2 pounds of Type A botulinum toxin, or 0.02 pounds of anthrax spores could each produce the same lethal effect per square-mile area.[85]

From a military perspective, inhalational anthrax is a particularly desirable bioweapon because it is essentially non-communicable.[86] A military could therefore use anthrax against another military without concern of secondary spread to the offensive military.[87] The offensive military could also employ known disease-mitigating agents such as the anthrax vaccine or antibiotics to protect service members when entering a

---

[82]COL Donald G. Curry Jr., ―The Case for _Forced' Health Protection" (U.S. Army War College Strategy Research Project, U.S. Army War College, 2004), 5, http://www.dtic.mil/cgi-bin/GetTRDoc?Location=U2&doc=GetTRDoc.pdf&AD= ADA424088 (accessed 27 October 2010).

[83]Davis and Johnson-Winegar, 22-23.

[84]Ibid., 23.

[85]Ibid.

[86]Ibid., 22.

[87]Ibid.

known, contaminated environment.[88] This force protection strategy confers both physical and psychological benefits for a military that might employ anthrax offensively.[89] Anthrax has a short incubation period of one to six days. This short incubation period would allow rapid, potent effects, desirable in an offensive weapon.[90]

Literature on nations with known and suspected bioweapons programs is incomplete. Details regarding specific offensive capabilities of individual states vary. However, it would not be unreasonable to assume that states with bioweapons capacities have explored or developed anthrax as a bioweapon within their arsenal.[91] According to Col (Dr.) Jim Davis and Dr. Anna Johnson-Winegar, states with former or current ability to use anthrax as a bioweapon include United States, the former Soviet Union, Israel, Taiwan, Libya, Iraq, Iran, Syria, Russia, and South Africa[92] According to biological terrorism expert Dr. Seth Carus, other states that may have bioweapons programs include Bulgaria, China, Cuba, Egypt, India, Laos, Libya, North Korea, Taiwan, and Vietnam.[93]

---

[88]Ibid.

[89]Ibid.

[90]Ibid., 22-23.

[91]Ibid., 23.

[92]Ibid., 23-24.

[93]Ibid., 24.

Anthrax Vaccine

The original human anthrax vaccine was developed in the 1950s.[94] The vaccine manufacturing process changed following a 1962 study on the vaccine's use in mill workers, and the Michigan Department of Public Health (MDPH) began producing the vaccine.[95] The Division of Biologics, National Institutes of Health licensed the MDPH vaccine in 1970.[96] In 1995, MDPH changed its name to the Michigan Biologic Products Institute.[97] In January 1998, the Michigan Biologics Products Institute halted anthrax vaccine production to renovate the production facility.[98] The facility was sold to the BioPort Corporation in September 1998.[99] In December 2001, the FDA approved BioPort's AVA manufacturing facility. In January 2002, the FDA allowed the BioPort Corporation to begin distribution of the AVA.[100]

---

[94]United States General Accounting Office, GAO/T-NSIAD-99-148, *Safety and Efficacy of the Anthrax Vaccine* (Washington, DC: Government Printing Office, 29 April 1999), 4.

[95]Ibid.

[96]Ibid.

[97]Ibid., 3.

[98]United States Food and Drug Administration, Bioterrorism and Drug Preparedness, ―FDA Approves License Supplements For Anthrax Vaccine,‖ http://www.fda.gov/Drugs/EmergencyPreparedness/BioterrorismandDrugPreparedness/ucm133146.htm (accessed 12 September 2010).

[99]Ibid.

[100]Ibid.

The AVA was developed from an attenuated strain of *B. anthracis*.[101] The AVA derives from the cell-free culture filtrate of this attenuated strain (V770-NP1-R) adsorbed onto an aluminum salt.[102] The AVA is indicated for people between 18 and 65 years at high risk of exposure to anthrax.[103] Although AVA's mechanism of protection is not known, antibodies against PA may contribute to disease protection by neutralizing PA activities, and therefore limiting the effects of LF or EF.[104] Adult vaccination with the AVA induces an immune response measured by indirect hemagglutination in 83 percent of vaccinees two weeks after the first dose and in 91 percent of vaccinees who receive two or more doses.[105] Approximately 95 percent of vaccinated individuals demonstrate a fourfold rise in anti-PA immunoglobulin G titers after three AVA doses.[106] Increased antibody levels are suggestive of protection against disease; however, there is no precise level at which protection is assured.

The originally-licensed anthrax vaccine included six doses administered within the first 18 months, and subsequent annual boosters. In December 2008, the FDA

---

[101]United States Food and Drug Administration, Vaccines, Blood and Biologics, ―Anthrax,‖ http://www.fda.gov/biologicsbloodvaccines/vaccines/ucm061751.htm (accessed 28 October 2010).

[102]Ibid.; Advisory Committee on Immunization Practices, ―Use of Anthrax Vaccine in the United States,‖ 5.

[103]Emergent BioSolutions, ―BioThrax® (Anthrax Vaccine Adsorbed).‖

[104]Ibid.

[105]Advisory Committee on Immunization Practices, ―Use of Anthrax Vaccine in the United States,‖ 7.

[106]Ibid.

approved a change to a five dose regimen for the primary series, with subsequent annual boosters.[107]

Anthrax Vaccine Efficacy

AVA efficacy data include animal studies, human studies, and immunogenicity data in both mammals and humans.[108] "The protective efficacy of the alum-precipitated vaccine (the original form of the PA filtrate vaccine) and AVA (adsorbed to aluminum hydroxide) have been demonstrated in several animal models using different routes of administration."[109] The AVA vaccine protects against pulmonary challenge in Rhesus monkeys, using a limited number of *B. anthracis* strains.[110]

Between 1955 and 1959 a controlled human study was conducted on the human anthrax vaccine developed in the 1950s.[111] This study included 1,249 millworkers with occupational exposure to animal hides.[112] Three hundred seventy nine study participants received the anthrax vaccine, 414 received a placebo, 116 received an incomplete vaccination series of either vaccine or placebo, and 340 did not receive treatment.[113] Prior to the study, the annual number of human anthrax cases (inhalational and cutaneous)

---

[107]Emergent BioSolutions, "BioThrax® (Anthrax Vaccine Adsorbed)."

[108]Advisory Committee on Immunization Practices, "Use of Anthrax Vaccine in the United States," 7.

[109]Ibid.

[110]Ibid.

[111]Emergent BioSolutions, "BioThrax® (Anthrax Vaccine Adsorbed).

[112]Ibid.

[113]Ibid.

among the study population was 1.2 cases per 100 employees. During the vaccine trial, five inhalation and 21 cutaneous anthrax cases were reported.[114] Of the five cases of inhalational anthrax, two patients received placebo vaccines and three patients were in the observational group.[115] Of the 21 patients with cutaneous disease, 15 had received placebo, three had received no vaccine, and three had received an incomplete anthrax vaccine series.[116] Of the three patients with cutaneous disease who had received prior anthrax vaccine, one patient became ill immediately prior to the third scheduled dose, one case occurred 13 months after the third of six planned doses, and one case occurred prior the fourth scheduled dose.[117] Based upon the frequency of both inhalational and cutaneous anthrax, the demonstrated efficacy of the vaccine to prevent all types of anthrax disease was 92.5 percent.[118]

The CDC collected data on the occurrence of anthrax disease in persons working in or living near mills in the United States between 1962 and 1974.[119] During this time period anthrax vaccination among mill workers was common, but was not universal. Of the 27 cases of anthrax identified by the CDC in this 12 year interval, 24 cases occurred in unvaccinated patients.[120] In the three cases identified in which the patient had received

---

[114]Ibid.

[115]Ibid.

[116]Ibid.

[117]Ibid.

[118]Ibid.

[119]Ibid.

[120]Ibid.

prior anthrax vaccine, one case occurred after one dose of vaccine, and two cases occurred in patients who had received two doses of vaccine.[121] No disease cases were reported in individuals who had received at least three of the six recommended anthrax vaccine doses.[122]

Safety

In a five-year safety study of 15,907 doses of anthrax vaccine administered by the subcutaneous route to approximately 7,000 textile workers, laboratory workers, and other at-risk individuals, mild local reactions were the most common reported adverse reactions.[123] Twenty four patients (0.15 percent of vaccine doses administered) reported severe local reactions defined as skin erythema or induration over 120 mm in diameter, or associated with limitation of arm motion or axillary lymph node tenderness.[124] One hundred fifty patients (0.94 percent of vaccine doses administered) reported moderate local reactions defined as skin edema or induration between 30 and 120 mm in diameter.[125] One thousand three hundred seventy three patients (8.63 percent of vaccine doses administered) reported mild local reactions defined as only erythema or induration less than 30 mm in diameter.[126] Four patients (<0.06 percent of vaccine doses

---

[121]Ibid.

[122]Ibid.

[123]Ibid.

[124]Ibid.

[125]Ibid.

[126]Ibid.

administered) experienced systemic reactions including transient fever, chills, nausea, and general body aches.[127]

The DoD has assessed adverse events in association with the AVIP in two large studies. Between September and October 1998, patients in Korea completed a mandatory self-administered questionnaire in association with planned anthrax vaccines.[128] The questionnaire included information on the patient's health status, medication use, and queried reactions to any prior dose(s) of anthrax vaccine.[129] Data from 6,879 questionnaires were reviewed: 37 percent (2531) of respondents were receiving their first dose of anthrax vaccine, 63 percent had received one (2427 respondents) or two (1921 respondents) prior AVA doses.[130] Female service members reported more adverse events associated with their prior vaccinations(s) than did male service members. Both men and women most frequently reported adverse events that were localized, self-limited, and minor.[131] Eighty two of the 4348 patients (1.9 percent) who had received a prior anthrax vaccine dose reported some limitation in their work performance or that they were placed on limited duty in association with vaccination, 13 patients (0.3 percent) reported less

---

[127]Ibid.

[128]Centers for Disease Control and Prevention, ─Surveillance for Adverse Events Associated with Anthrax Vaccination-U.S. Department of Defense, 1998–2000," *MMWR Recommendations and Reports* 49, no 16 (28 April 2000): 341.

[129]Ibid.

[130]Ibid.

[131]Ibid., 342.

than or equal to one day lost from work, 21 (0.5 percent) requested clinical evaluation, and one patient (0.02 percent) was hospitalized for an injection site reaction.[132]

In 1998, Tripler Army Medical Center surveyed 603 United States military health care workers in the Korea Medical Augmentee Program.[133] Study participants completed a self-administered questionnaire regarding adverse events associated with anthrax vaccination. Data collection for approximately 80 percent of the initial study patients (479) was completed through the fourth AVA dose.[134] ―After the first anthrax dose, 47 (7.9 percent) of 595 reported seeking medical advice and/or taking time off work for a complaint (e.g., muscle or joint aches, headache, or fatigue); after the second dose, 30 (5.1 percent) of 585; after the third dose, 16 (3.0 percent) of 536; and after the fourth dose, 17 (3.1 percent) of 536.‖[135]

In addition to the studies described above, the DoD uses the Vaccine Adverse Event Reporting System (VAERS) to report adverse events potentially related to any vaccination. VAERS, managed jointly by the CDC and FDA, is a surveillance system for recognizing vaccine adverse events not apparent in pre-licensure clinical trials, monitoring known vaccine adverse reactions, identifying possible risk factors, and vaccine lot surveillance.[136] VAERS was established in 1990, and receives approximately

---

[132]Ibid.

[133]Ibid.

[134]Ibid., 343.

[135]Ibid.

[136]United States Food and Drug Administration, ―Review of VAERS Anthrax Vaccine Reports Received through 8/15/05, and Adverse Event Reports Submitted to

15,000 vaccine adverse event reports annually.[137] Vaccine manufacturers, health care

providers, patients, caregivers, attorneys, and interested parties submit VAERS reports.

VAERS is limited because it is a passive surveillance system. However, adverse events

may be linked to specific vaccines when patterns of clinical or demographic data emerge.

The Defense Medical Surveillance System (DMSS) consolidates VAERS reports

related to anthrax vaccinations.[138] From 1990 through 31 March 2005, approximately 1.3

million service members received 5.3 million doses of AVA, and 4,279 VAERS reports

were submitted.[139] Based on pattern assessments of this data, descriptive analyses, data

mining, and queries of specific clinical conditions with known incidence rates and risk

intervals, the FDA did not conclude that a causal relationship exists between serious

adverse events and administration of AVA.[140]

Between 2002 and 2008, the CDC sponsored a prospective double-blinded,

randomized, placebo-controlled study to evaluate the impact on vaccine safety and

immune response of a change in anthrax vaccine administration route from subcutaneous

to intramuscular, and a reduced number of vaccine doses.[141] This six year study included

---

Docket No. 1980N-0208," 2, http://www.anthrax.mil/documents/965VAERSvol225.pdf
(accessed 9 November 2010).

[137]Ibid.

[138]Centers for Disease Control and Prevention, –Surveillance for Adverse Events
Associated with Anthrax Vaccination-U.S. Department of Defense, 1998–2000," 343.

[139]United States Food and Drug Administration, –Review of VAERS Anthrax
Vaccine Reports Received through 8/15/05, and Adverse Event Reports Submitted to
Docket No. 1980N-0208," 8.

[140]Ibid., 9.

[141]Emergent BioSolutions, –BioThrax® (Anthrax Vaccine Adsorbed)."

1,564 healthy volunteers.[142] Study subjects completed a 14-day post-vaccination diary card after the first two vaccine doses and a 28-day post-vaccination diary card after the subsequent doses.[143] Adverse reaction data were collected from diary cards and clinical exams performed prior to and following each injection, at one to three days after each injection, and at 28 days after the third and fourth injections.[144] Less than one percent of vaccinees experienced severe adverse reactions.[145] Vaccinations administered by the intramuscular route as compared to the subcutaneous route demonstrated both decreased quantity and duration of local reactions to include warmth, tenderness, itching, erythema, induration, edema, and nodules.[146] In this study, women again reported more injection-site adverse reactions than did men.[147] Women also reported more vaccine-associated systemic adverse reactions than men such as fatigue, muscle aches, and headache.[148]

The majority of study participants reported a brief local pain or burning sensation with vaccine injection.[149] Study participants rated injection site pain on a scale of 0-10.[150] Forty one percent of participants described the pain as a score greater than three

---

[142]Ibid.

[143]Ibid.

[144]Ibid.

[145]Ibid.

[146]Ibid.

[147]Ibid.

[148]Ibid.

[149]Ibid.

[150]Ibid.

following subcutaneous injection, while 26 percent of patients reported the pain as a score greater than three following intramuscular injection.[151] The majority of serious adverse reactions reported during the study were not related to vaccination.[152] Two serious adverse reactions possibly related to anthrax vaccination occurred during the study: a case of anaphylaxis and a case of an autoimmune disorder.[153] Of the 44 pregnant patients who received the anthrax vaccine, the majority delivered healthy term infants.[154]

Two additional studies have queried the health of pregnancies and infants in association with anthrax vaccine. A cohort study, based on computerized records, of women between 17 and 44 years of age stationed at either Fort Stewart or Hunter Army Airfield Georgia between January 1999 and March 2000 evaluated pregnancy rates, fetal loss, and adverse birth outcomes among women who had received the anthrax vaccine.[155] Of the 4,092 women studied, 3,136 women received at least one dose of anthrax vaccine.[156] Five hundred thirteen pregnancies occurred, of which 385 pregnancies occurred following one or more doses of anthrax vaccine.[157] The pregnancy rate ratio

---

[151]Ibid.

[152]Ibid.

[153]Ibid.

[154]Ibid.

[155]Andrew R. Wiesen and Christopher L. Littell, ―Relationship Between Prepregnancy Anthrax Vaccination and Pregnancy and Birth Outcomes Among US Army Women,‖ *Journal of the American Medical Association* 287, no. 12 (27 March 2002): 1556.

[156]Ibid.

[157]Ibid.

comparing vaccinated with unvaccinated women was 0.94 (95 percent confidence interval, 0.8-1.2; P=.60).[158] Three hundred fifty three live births were known, while 25 pregnancies were lost to follow-up.[159] Although the study did not have sufficient power to detect adverse birth outcomes, the observed infant structural abnormality rate was consistent with national rates, and the percentage of low-birth-weight infants was approximately half of the national rate.[160] The authors concluded that ―These results do not support the hypothesis of a decrease in pregnancy rates nor an increase in fetal loss rates or adverse fetal outcome among those receiving anthrax vaccination prior to pregnancy.‖[161]

A subsequent retrospective cohort study published in 2008 evaluated birth defects among all babies born to United States female service members between 1998 and 2004.[162] The study utilized multivariable regression models to query potential associations between maternal anthrax vaccination and birth defects in live born infants.[163] Service members delivered 115,169 infants during this six year period, 37,140 infants were born to women who had ever received the anthrax vaccine, and 3,465 infants

---

[158]Ibid.

[159]Ibid.

[160]Ibid., 1559.

[161]Ibid.

[162]Margaret A. K. Ryan et al., ―Birth Defects Among Infants Born to Women Who Received Anthrax Vaccine In Pregnancy,‖ *American Journal of Epidemiology* 168, no. 4 (2 July 2008): 434.

[163]Ibid.

were born to women vaccinated in the first trimester of pregnancy.[164] Birth defects were slightly more common infants exposed to anthrax vaccine in the first trimester as compared to infants exposed to anthrax vaccine in the second and third trimesters (odds ratio of 1.18, 95 percent confidence interval: 0.997, 1.41). However, the authors concluded that this small increase —was not statistically significant when compared with that of infants born to women vaccinated outside of pregnancy.‖[165]

Women who were vaccinated prior to pregnancy or in the second or third trimesters of pregnancy did not have an increased risk of delivering an infant with a birth defect compared with non-vaccinated women.[166] The authors concluded that —There are several possible explanations for any observed association with first trimester exposures not being causal and, in fact, the degree of association observed here might be expected in any cohort of late-recognized pregnancies. Nonetheless, a causative association cannot be completely ruled out.‖[167] The authors interpret their analysis as reassuring in the event of an inadvertent vaccination during pregnancy, but suggest that women who do not have a known risk of anthrax should continue to avoid vaccination during pregnancy.[168] This guidance is consistent with multiple ACIP vaccine recommendations which suggest careful assessment of exposure risks prior to administration of vaccinations during pregnancy.

---

[164]Ibid.

[165]Ibid., 440.

[166]Ibid.

[167]Ibid.

[168]Ibid.

History of AVIP Policy

In December 1997, the Secretary of Defense approved the AVIP contingent on four conditions: supplemental vaccine testing, a reliable immunization tracking system, approved plans for implementation and communication, and independent medical review of the AVIP.[169] In May 1998, the Secretary of Defense recommended implementation of the AVIP for the total force.[170] In March 1999, Under Secretary of Defense Rudolph F. de Leon expanded the AVIP to include immediate application for all U.S. military personnel, essential DoD, and essential contractor personnel assigned in Southwest Asia (Kuwait, Saudi Arabia, Bahrain, Jordan, Qatar, Oman, United Arab Emirates, Yemen, and Israel) and the Korean Peninsula for any period of time.[171]

In July 2000, Deputy Secretary of Defense Rudolph F. de Leon directed a slowed execution of the AVIP in response to a shortage of available vaccine associated with lack of production.[172] In contrast to the previous ―one day" policy, personnel assigned or deployed to Southwest Asia or the Korean Peninsula for at least 30 days were directed to receive anthrax vaccine commencing 45 days prior to deployment.[173] Routine

---

[169]Secretary of Defense, *Implementation of the Anthrax Vaccination Program for the Total Force*, Memorandum (Washington, DC: Secretary of Defense, 18 May 1998).

[170]Ibid.

[171]Under Secretary of Defense, *Change to Anthrax Vaccine Immunization Program (AVIP) Operational Procedure (One Day Policy)*, Memorandum (Washington, DC: Under Secretary of Defense, 30 March 1999).

[172]Deputy Secretary of Defense, *Temporary Slowing and Future Resumption of Anthrax Vaccine Immunization Program (AVIP)*, Memorandum (Washington, DC: Deputy Secretary of Defense, 17 July 2000).

[173]Ibid.

vaccinations in non-deploying personnel were deferred to ensure supply to personnel deploying to Southwest Asia or the Korean Peninsula.[174] In November 2000, due to ongoing vaccine shortage, the Deputy Secretary of Defense redefined execution of the AVIP to include only personnel assigned to Southwest Asia for 30 days or more.[175]

With an ongoing vaccine shortage, in June 2001 the Deputy Secretary of Defense further amended AVIP implementation to include only personnel involved in designated special mission units, vaccine manufacturing, and research.[176] In June 2002, following FDA approval of the renovated anthrax manufacturing facility, the Deputy Secretary of Defense reintroduced the AVIP.[177] The plan for re-inception included military personnel and essential emergency civilians and contractors assigned to high-risk areas for more than 15 days.[178] In June 2004, the AVIP scope expanded to include service members, essential contractors, and civilians deploying to the Korean Peninsula for 15 days or longer, all uniformed personnel serving in the Central Command Area of Responsibility,

---

[174]Ibid.

[175]Deputy Secretary of Defense, *Additional Temporary Slowing and Future Resumption of Anthrax Vaccine Immunization Program (AVIP)*, Memorandum (Washington, DC: Deputy Secretary of Defense, 27 November 2000).

[176]Secretary of The Army, *Slowdown of the Anthrax Vaccine Immunization Program (AVIP)*, Memorandum (Washington, DC: Secretary of The Army, 8 June 2001).

[177]Deputy Secretary of Defense, *Reintroduction of the Anthrax Vaccine Immunization Program (AVIP)*, Memorandum (Washington, DC: Deputy Secretary of Defense, 28 June 2002).

[178]Ibid.

and voluntary anthrax vaccine administration for family members of personnel living in Korea.[179]

Between 1998 and December 2003, the DoD administered the anthrax vaccine to more than one million military, civilian, and contractor personnel.[180] On 23 December 2003, the United States District Court for the District of Columbia issued a preliminary injunction against the operation of the AVIP.[181] In response, Deputy Secretary of Defense David S. C. Chu halted all anthrax immunizations. The Army service message published on 24 December 2003 regarding the injunction specified that the ―focus of the legal ruling is whether the vaccine is properly licensed for use against inhalation anthrax (not cutaneous or gastrointestinal), and not whether the vaccine is considered safe.‖[182]

On 29 December 2003, the FDA published a *Federal Register* notice detailing its intent to affirm the vaccine‛s approval for anthrax disease, independent of exposure route.[183] In the December 2003 notice, the FDA acknowledged that the 1950s clinical data included too few cases of inhalational anthrax to clearly demonstrate that AVA

---

[179]Ibid.

[180]Department of the Army, *Temporarily Stop Giving Anthrax Immunizations to All DOD Personnel*, All Army Activities Message (Washington, DC: Department of the Army, 24 December 2003).

[181]Under Secretary of Defense, *Anthrax Vaccine Immunization Program*, Memorandum (Washington, DC: Under Secretary of Defense, 23 December 2003).

[182]Department of the Army, *Temporarily Stop Giving Anthrax Immunizations to All DOD Personnel*.

[183]Robert Roos, ―FDA Seeks Comments on Controversial Anthrax Vaccine,‖ Center for Infectious Disease Research and Policy Academic Health Center, University of Minnesota, http://www.cidrap.umn.edu/cidrap/content/bt/anthrax/news/ jan1305anthrax.html (accessed 11 November 2010).

prevented inhalational anthrax.[184] However, the FDA did emphasize that the 1950s

clinical data demonstrated 92.5 percent vaccine efficacy against all types of anthrax

disease.[185] On 7 January 2004, the United States District Court for the District of

Columbia issued a stay of the December 2003 injunction.[186] The Under Secretary of

Defense directed immediate resumption of the AVIP on 7 January 2004.[187]

On 27 October 2004, the United States District Court for the District of Columbia

again issued an injunction against the operation of the AVIP.[188] The October 2004

injunction was based on a decision by the Court that the FDA was required to solicit

additional public comments prior to finalizing the conclusion that anthrax vaccine is safe

and effective for the prevention of inhalational anthrax.[189] US District Judge Emmet G.

Sullivan found that the FDA had failed to follow its own policies by not soliciting public

comments before confirming (in December 2003) that AVA was approved for prevention

of all forms of anthrax.[190] In December 1985 when a FDA expert panel recommended

confirmation of continued licensure of the AVA, the FDA gave the public 90 days to

---

[184]Ibid.

[185]Ibid.

[186]Under Secretary of Defense, *Anthrax Vaccine Immunization Program Resumption*, Memorandum (Washington, DC: Under Secretary of Defense,7 January 2004).

[187]Ibid.

[188]Ibid.

[189]Ibid.

[190]Roos. ―FDA Seeks Comments on Controversial Anthrax Vaccine.‖

comment on vaccine approval.[191] According to Sullivan in October 2004, the FDA never

confirmed AVA licensing for all routes of anthrax exposure following the December

2003 ruling.[192] Additionally, according to Sullivan, the FDA's December 2003 ruling

relied on post-1985 research findings, without opportunity for public comment.[193]

In response to the Court injunction, the DoD again halted all anthrax vaccinations

on 27 October 2004.[194] On 27 January 2005, the FDA issued an Emergency Use

Authorization (EUA) to allow the DoD to resume anthrax vaccinations, with the

condition that vaccine recipients would have the option to refuse the vaccine.[195] In April

2005, the District Court modified the 27 October 2004 injunction to allow anthrax

vaccines administration under the EUA.[196] Under the EUA, the DoD provided eligible

service members with information about the AVIP, and encouraged vaccination, but

neither ordered nor required vaccination.[197] The scope of the AVIP included personnel

serving in Central Command for 15 or more consecutive days, with United States forces

in Korea for 15 or more consecutive days, and other categories of personnel subject to

---

[191]Ibid.

[192]Ibid.

[193]Ibid.

[194]Secretary of Defense, *Anthrax Vaccine Immunization Program Pause*, Memorandum (Washington, DC: Secretary of Defense, 27 October 2004).

[195]Deputy Secretary of Defense, *Resumption of the Anthrax Vaccine Immunization Program (AVIP) Under Emergency Use Authorization (EUA)*, Memorandum (Washington, DC: Deputy Secretary of Defense, 25 April 2005).

[196]Ibid.

[197]Ibid.

mandatory vaccination prior to 27 October 2004.[198] Under the EUA, personnel who had

started the anthrax vaccine series but were no longer at heightened exposure risk were not

eligible for additional doses in the series or to receive annual booster doses.[199]

On 15 December 2005, the FDA issued a Final Rule and Final Order on the status

of the AVA.[200] Following review of scientific evidence and public comment, the FDA

licensed AVA for the prevention of anthrax disease through all routes of exposure.[201]

This regulatory action removed the need for an EUA.[202] Following this ruling, in late

December 2005, the DoD elected to continue implementation of the AVIP as authorized

in April 2005 to include eligibility of select personnel for vaccination, with the continued

option to refuse the vaccine.[203]

In October 2006, the DoD announced plans to resume mandatory anthrax

vaccination for personnel assigned to high-threat areas and personnel with special

mission roles such as biowarfare and bioterrorism response.[204] This transition was

consistent with the December 2005 FDA ruling, which stated:

---

[198]Ibid.

[199]Ibid.

[200]Assistant Secretary of Defense, *Continuation of the Anthrax Vaccine Immunization Program (AVIP)*, Memorandum (Washington, DC: Department of Defense, 22 December 2005).

[201]Ibid.

[202]Ibid.

[203]Ibid.

[204]Deputy Secretary of Defense, *Anthrax Vaccine Immunization Program (AVIP)*, Memorandum (Washington, DC: Deputy Secretary of Defense 12 October 2006).

Based on the continuing heightened threat to some U.S. personnel of attack with anthrax spores, the Department of Defense will resume a mandatory Anthrax Vaccine Immunization Program, consistent with Food and Drug Administration guidelines and the best practice of medicine, for designated military personnel, emergency-essential and comparable Department of Defense civilian employees, and certain contractor personnel performing essential services.[205]

This plan did not involve a shift in the patient population targeted for vaccination.

In December 2006, the Under Secretary of Defense detailed instructions for resumption of the mandatory AVIP.[206] In the absence of a medical or administrative exemption, mandatory anthrax vaccines are required for uniformed personnel assigned to the Central Command area of responsibility for 15 or more consecutive days, uniformed personnel assigned to the Korean Peninsula for 15 or more consecutive days, emergency-essential DoD civilian and contractor personnel assigned to Central Command or the Korean Peninsula for 15 or more consecutive days, and other previously-designated specified high risk groups.[207] Personnel eligible for voluntary vaccination include civilian employees and contractors assigned for 15 or more consecutive days to Central Command and Korea not designated as essential or emergency personnel, adult family members accompanying military, civilian, and contractor personnel for 15 or more consecutive days to Central Command or Korea, vaccine manufacturing and research personnel on a case-by-case basis, and individuals not subject to mandatory vaccination who have received at least one prior vaccine dose and desire to continue the dosing

---

[205]Ibid.

[206]Under Secretary of Defense, *Implementation of the Anthrax Vaccine Immunization Program (AVIP)*, Memorandum (Washington, DC: Under Secretary of Defense, 6 December 2006).

[207]Ibid.

series.[208] Personnel may begin immunizations up to 60 days prior to deployment, with a goal of at least three vaccine doses prior to deployment.[209] In accordance with this guidance, each service was required to submit and receive approval for a service-specific AVIP implementation plan prior to re-inception of immunizations. In early February 2007, each service-specific policy was approved.

Current AVIP Policy

With exception of medical or administrative contraindications, anthrax vaccination is mandatory for service members, emergency essential civilian employees and contractors deployed to United States Central Command or Korea areas of responsibility for 15 or more consecutive days.[210] Anthrax vaccinations are also mandatory for certain service members assigned to units with specific high-risk functions such as biodefense missions.[211] Following a 2008 study, the current FDA-licensed anthrax dosing schedule is five doses administered at time zero, four weeks, six months, 12 months, and 18 months, plus annual boosters given intramuscularly.[212]

Opinions Regarding AVIP Policy

Divergent opinions exist regarding the AVA and the AVIP. The Military Vaccine Agency (MILVAX) AVIP website includes the following statements: ―The anthrax

---

[208]Ibid.

[209]Ibid.

[210]Department of Defense, ―What You Need to Know About Anthrax Vaccine,‖ http://www.anthrax.mil/documents/1106AvipTrifold.pdf (accessed 4 November 2010).

[211]Ibid.

[212]Ibid.

vaccine is safe and effective." —The threat from anthrax is deadly and real." —Vaccination offers a layer of protection in addition to antibiotics and other measures needed for certain members of the Armed Forces."[213] In contrast, opponents view anthrax as an unclear threat, and suggest that viable non-vaccine alternative force protection measures exist.

Arguments and Evidence Cited by Proponents of the AVIP Policy

The FDA's Center for Biologics Evaluation and Research (CBER) regulates all licensed vaccines in the United States.[214] In addition to vigorous pre-licensing evaluation of a vaccine's ability to generate an immune response, safety, and efficacy; following licensure the CBER monitors all vaccines for safety, purity, and potency.[215] In addition to recent (2008) review by the FDA, seven independent civilian panels have evaluated the safety and efficacy of the anthrax vaccine since 1978.[216]

In 1972 responsibility for vaccine regulation shifted from the National Institutes of Health (NIH) to the FDA.[217] Concurrent with this transfer of responsibility, the FDA convened expert panels for every vaccine in use in the United States to determine

---

[213]Military Vaccine (MILVAX) Agency, —AVIP Anthrax Vaccine Immunization Program," http://www.anthrax.osd.mil/default.asp (accessed 7 November 2010).

[214]United States Food and Drug Administration, Vaccines, Blood, and Biologics, —Vaccine Product Approval Process," http://www.fda.gov/biologics bloodvaccines/developmentapprovalprocess/biologicslicenseapplicationsblaprocess/ucm1 33096.htm (accessed 11 November 2010).

[215]Ibid.

[216]Military Vaccine (MILVAX) Agency, —Anthrax Vaccine Immunization Program (AVIP) Questions and Answers," 11.

[217]Ibid., 16.

whether appropriate safety and efficacy data existed to support continued licensure.[218]

The Panel on Review of Bacterial Vaccines and Toxoids included infectious disease physicians and pharmaceutical manufacturing quality experts.[219] The Panel on Review of Bacterial Vaccines and Toxoids initially met in 1978 and published a report in the 1985. The panel concluded that AVA was safe, effective, not misbranded, and recommended continued vaccine licensure.[220]

The Defense Health Board (DHB), previously known as Armed Forces Epidemiological Board (AFEB), consists of civilian scientists and physicians who advise the Surgeons General of the Armed Services.[221] The DHB published the results of evaluations of the AVA in 1994, 1996, 1999, and 2000.[222] In 1994, the DHB concluded that the AVA was appropriate for personnel deploying to high-threat areas.[223] In 1996, the DHB endorsed the AVIP. In 1999, the DHB again affirmed support for the AVIP.[224] In 2000, the DHB stated:

> we are concerned and somewhat surprised at the criticism surrounding the program given the high level of professionalism that had characterized this effort.

---

[218]Ibid., 11-12.

[219]Ibid., 12.

[220]Kathryn C. Zoon, ―Vaccines, Pharmaceutical Products, and Bioterrorism: Challenges for the U.S. Food and Drug Administration," *Emerging Infectious Diseases* 5, no. 4 (July-August 1999): 536.

[221]Military Vaccine (MILVAX) Agency, ―Anthrax Vaccine Immunization Program Questions and Answers," 12.

[222]Ibid.

[223]Ibid.

[224]Ibid.

. . . Anthrax vaccine is a fully licensed FDA vaccine. The vaccine does cause local side effects, but has an excellent safety profile. The Anthrax Vaccine Immunization Program has carefully tabulated person-specific immunization data and has assiduously investigated reported complications associated with receipt of anthrax vaccine. These data have been regularly reviewed by the board and attest to the safety of the vaccine.[225]

Given the expertise and long experience of the DHB with the AVA, its continued support for the AVIP is of particular significance.

The Advisory Committee on Immunization Practices (ACIP) is a panel of prominent clinicians and scientists that advises the CDC and sets national standards for vaccine policy. In 2000, the Advisory Committee on Immunization Practices (ACIP) reviewed AVA safety and efficacy data.[226] The ACIP recommended routine anthrax vaccination for people employed in activities with a high potential for aerosol production of anthrax or employed in fields involving high quantities or concentrations of anthrax, but did not universally recommend routine preexposure vaccination against the threat of bioterrorism.

> Although groups initially considered for preexposure vaccination for bioterrorism preparedness included emergency first responders, federal responders, medical practitioners, and private citizens, vaccination of these groups is not recommended. Recommendations regarding preexposure vaccination should be based on a calculable risk assessment. At present, the target population for a bioterrorist release of *B. anthracis* cannot be predetermined, and the risk of exposure cannot be calculated. In addition, studies suggest an extremely low risk for exposure related to secondary aerosolization of previously settled *B. anthracis* spores. Because of these factors, preexposure vaccination for the above groups is not recommended. For the military and other select populations or for groups for

---

[225]Ibid.

[226]Advisory Committee on Immunization Practices, "Use of Anthrax Vaccine in the United States," 7.

which a calculable risk can be assessed, preexposure vaccination may be indicated.[227]

Although the 2000 ACIP recommendations did not explicitly endorse preexposure anthrax vaccine for military personnel, the recommendations did acknowledge the potential for increased exposure risk among the military population.

In 2002, following the bioterrorism events of 2001 in which *B. anthracis* spores were sent through the United States Postal Service, the ACIP released recommendations on using anthrax vaccine in response to terrorism.[228] In addition to reaffirming the recommendation for pre-exposure vaccination for persons with repeated exposure to *B. anthracis,* the ACIP endorsed availability of AVA as a 3-dose regimen in conjunction with antibiotics under an Investigational New Drug (IND) application with the FDA for unvaccinated persons at risk for inhalational anthrax.[229]

The 2010 ACIP recommendations included input from the ACIP Anthrax Vaccine Work Group, which convened in October 2007.[230] The ACIP Anthrax Vaccine Work Group includes representatives from the DoD, the American College of Occupational and Environmental Medicine, the InterAgency Board for Equipment Standardization and

---

[227]Ibid., 12.

[228]Advisory Committee on Immunization Practices, ―Notice to Readers: Use of Anthrax Vaccine in Response to Terrorism: Supplemental Recommendations of the Advisory Committee on Immunization Practices," *MMWR Recommendations and Reports* 51, no. 45 (15 November 2002): 1024.

[229]Ibid., 1025.

[230]Advisory Committee on Immunization Practices, ―Use of Anthrax Vaccine in the United States Recommendations of the Advisory Committee on Immunization Practices (ACIP), 2009," *MMWR Recommendations and Reports* 59, no. RR-6 (23 July 2010): 2.

Interoperability, the Office of the Biomedical Advanced Research and Development Authority, the National Institutes of Health (NIH), the American Veterinary Medical Association, the American Academy of Pediatrics, the American College of Obstetrics and Gynecology, the National Association of County and City Health Officials, and the Food and Drug Administration (FDA).[231] The 2010 ACIP recommendations directly address the potential benefits of pre-exposure AVA vaccination:

> By priming the immune system before exposure to *B. anthracis* spores, pre-event and preexposure vaccination might provide more protection than antimicrobial agents alone to persons at risk for occupational exposure to *B. anthracis,* including protection for persons exposed to large innocula, protection if the public health infrastructure cannot ensure immediate availability or timely delivery of post event antimicrobial agents, and potential benefits if bioengineered strains were released, limiting antimicrobial PEP effectiveness.[232]

In the 2010 recommendations, the ACIP continues to recommend a calculated risk assessment for use of pre-exposure vaccine.[233]

The Cochrane Collaboration is an international organization that produces systematic reviews of the medical literature on specific topics.[234] Cochrane reviews assemble primary literature, and provide evidence-based answers to challenging questions.[235] In a 2008 review of available randomized controlled trials of anthrax vaccines, the authors found that a large cluster randomized controlled trial of an anthrax

---

[231]Ibid.

[232]Ibid., 18.

[233]Ibid., 19.

[234]The Cochrane Collaboration, ―Cochrane Reviews,‖ http://www.cochrane.org/cochrane-reviews (accessed 11 November 2010).

[235]Ibid.

vaccine used in the former Soviet Union was effective at preventing cutnaeous anthrax. Further, "More recent types of vaccines tested in the smaller trials, also based on inactivated components of the anthrax bacterium, appear to have few adverse events and to stimulate a good immune response."[236]

In 2000, the United States Congress directed the DoD to support an independent review of the AVA by the IOM.[237] The Committee to Assess the Safety and Efficacy of the Anthrax Vaccine reviewed data; heard testimony from federal agencies, the AVA manufacturer, research scientists, and from persons with concerns about the safety or efficacy of the vaccine.[238] The 2002 IOM report concluded that the AVA was both safe and effective. As indicated by evidence from studies in both humans and animals, the committee concluded that AVA, as licensed, is an effective vaccine to protect humans against anthrax, including inhalational anthrax.

> Moreover, because the vaccine exerts its protection via an antigen crucial to the action of the bacterium's toxins, AVA should be effective against anthrax toxicity from all known strains of *B. anthracis,* as well as from any potential bioengineered strains. After examining data from numerous case reports and especially epidemiologic studies, the committee also concluded that AVA is reasonably safe. Within hours or days following vaccination, it is fairly common for recipients to experience some local events (e.g., redness, itching, swelling, or tenderness at the injection site); while a smaller number of vaccine recipients experience some systemic events (e.g., fever and malaise). But these immediate

---

[236]S. Donegan, R. Bellamy, and C. L. Gamble, ―Vaccines for Preventing Anthrax," Cochrane Database of Systematic Reviews 2009, Issue 2. Art. No: CD006403. DOI: 10.1002/14651858.CD006403.pub2, http://www2.cochrane.org/ reviews/en/ ab006403.html (accessed 20 March 2011).

[237]Committee to Assess the Safety and Efficacy of the Anthrax Vaccine and Medical Follow-Up Agency, 34.

[238]Ibid., 2.

reactions, and the rates at which they occur, are comparable to those observed with other vaccines regularly administered to adults.[239]

The IOM further reviewed AVA's manufacturing process, and found it to be consistent with the current FDA requirements.[240] In 2002, The IOM called for further ongoing monitoring of the AVA, and studies to quantify protective antibody levels.[241]

The Working Group on Civilian Bio-defense reviewed the all available anthrax literature in the late 1990s, and again in 2002.[242] The Working Group on Civilian Bio-defense included 23 experts from major academic medical centers, researchers, government, military, public health, and emergency management institutions and agencies.[243] The Working Group on Civilian Bio-defense concurred with the IOM report on the safety and efficacy of AVA.[244] In 1998, the US Department of Health and Human Services (DHHS) formed the Anthrax Vaccine Expert Committee (AVEC) to review VAERS reports involving anthrax vaccine.[245] The committee includes civilian physicians of various disciplines to include immunology, microbiology, neurology, rheumatology,

---

[239]Ibid.

[240]Ibid.

[241]Ibid.

[242]Military Vaccine (MILVAX) Agency, ―Anthrax Vaccine Immunization Program Questions and Answers," 13.

[243]Ibid.

[244]Ibid.

[245]Ibid., 14.

and internal medicine.[246] The AVEC has found no unexpected patterns in reported adverse events that are temporally related to the anthrax vaccine.[247]

Arguments and Evidence Cited by Opponents of the AVIP Policy

Opponents of the AVIP policy frequently cite several concerns regarding both the AVA and the AVIP. Concerns include safety and efficacy, manufacturing irregularities, indications for vaccine use, development of anthrax strains that are resistant to vaccination, and adverse events experienced by vaccinated patients. Vocal AVIP opponents include Dr. Meryl Nass, an Internal Medicine physician in Maine.[248]

Dr. Nass maintains a blog, anthraxvaccine.blogspot.com and a website www.anthraxvaccine.org. Both sites include extensive commentary regarding the anthrax vaccine. In a 2007 posting, Dr. Nass argues that military physicians are reluctant to report adverse events associated with the anthrax vaccine secondary to adverse career consequences, that VAERS reports demonstrate an increased rate of Gulf War Illness symptoms in anthrax vaccine recipients, that the Vaccine Healthcare Center (VHC) Network established in 2001 for monitoring of vaccine adverse events and research has failed to provide case-specific information to other physicians and the public, and that the design of several anthrax vaccine surveillance studies has been flawed.[249] In a 2002

---

[246]Ibid.

[247]Ibid.

[248]Meryl Nass, ―The Anthrax Vaccine Program: An Analysis of the CDC‗s Recommendations for Vaccine Use," *American Journal of Public Health* 92, no. 5 (May 2002): 719.

[249]Meryl Nass, ―Surveillance Program for Short-Term Health Effects of AVA," http://www.anthraxvaccine.org/NassDOD.htm (accessed 12 November 2010).

American Journal of Public Health article, she contends that the anthrax vaccine was never proven to be safe and effective, is one cause of Gulf War illness, and that vaccine production has been substandard.[250]

In 1998, Air Force Lieutenant Colonel Thomas Rempfer and a colleague actively pursued concerns that he and other unit members had about the AVA's efficacy.[251] Following review, Lt Col Rempfer refused to be vaccinated, and was disciplined.[252] Lt Col Rempfer has since testified before Congress regarding the AVIP, and brought suit against the FDA, the DHHS, and the DoD challenging the FDA's Final Order.[253] In his 2009 thesis entitled —Anthrax Vaccine as a Component of the Strategic National Stockpile: A Dilemma for Homeland Security," Lt Col Rempfer argues that the anthrax vaccine was —invented, patented, licensed, procured, altered, and mandated for decades almost exclusively by the military for a captive audience—soldiers."[254] Lt Col Rempfer

---

[250]Meryl Nass, —The Anthrax Vaccine Program: An Analysis of the CDC's Recommendations for Vaccine Use," 718.

[251]William H. McMichael, —Review Ordered for Anthrax Vaccine Refusers," *Army Times*, 26 April 2008, http://www.armytimes.com/news/2008/04/ SATURDAYmilitary_anthraxvaccines_042608w/ (accessed 12 November 2010).

[252]Ibid.

[253]United States District Court for the District of Columbia, Civil Action No. 06-2131, *Thomas Rempfer, et al., v. Andrew C. Von Eschenbach, Commissioner Food and Drug Administration, et al.*, http://www.anthrax.mil/documents/library/AnthraxAppeal Dismissal.pdf (accessed 12 November 2010).

[254]Thomas L. Rempfer, —Anthrax Vaccine as a Component of the Strategic National Stockpile: A Dilemma for Homeland Security" (Master's thesis, Naval Postgraduate School, Monterey, California, 2009), xix, https://www.hsdl.org/ homesec/docs/theses/09Dec_Rempfer.pdf (accessed 12 November 2010).

cites concerns with the AVIP to include AVA efficacy, manufacturing deviations, and association with Gulf War illness.[255]

In a 2009 article in the journal *Homeland Security Affairs,* Lt Col Rempfer argues that inconsistencies in DoD policies, safety and efficacy concerns, potency and quality control failures, poor threat assessments, and legal issues severely limit the AVIP.[256] Rempfer specifically questions the relationship of the 2001 bioterrorist attacks in the United States to the AVIP.

> The fact that the 2001 anthrax letter attacks were undertaken by the scientist in charge of vaccine potency testing for a program on the verge of failure, and that the attacks served to reinvigorate a troubled program in response to a —manufactured" crisis, creates fundamental doubts about expanding use of the vaccine.[257]

Rempfer argues for alternate anthrax threat countermeasures to include research, storage and security of pathogens, and new vaccine development.

Conclusion

This chapter provided the clinical, scientific, and historical framework necessary to understand the evolution of the AVIP program. An overview of vaccine efficacy and safety data, the history of DoD policy, current DoD AVIP policy, and divergent opinions surrounding the AVIP are essential for evaluation of the current AVIP. This literature review presented this information, organized into 12 sections. The following chapter will outline the methodology used to answer the research question.

---

[255]Ibid., xx.

[256]Thomas L. Rempfer, —The Anthrax Vaccine: A Dilemma for Homeland Security," *Homeland Security Affairs* 5, no. 2 (May 2009): 1.

[257]Ibid., 6.

CHAPTER 3

METHODOLOGY

The DoD must provide U.S. forces with reasonable levels of protection against
battle and nonbattle threats to health and well-being.
— Military Vaccine (MILVAX) Agency,
"Information About the Anthrax Vaccine and the AVIP"

Introduction

This chapter will outline the research methodology utilized to answer the thesis

research question. As previously introduced, the research question is: Based on available

evidence-based literature, what are the current known risks and benefits of the AVIP? For

the purposes of this study, risk is defined as the probability of harm (physical,

psychological, social, or economic) occurring in association with an intervention.

Probability and magnitude of possible harm may vary from minimal to significant.[258]

Benefit is defined as a desired outcome; an advantageous outcome.[259]

This study is qualitative and descriptive in nature. Strengths and limitations of this

research method are outlined in the current chapter. Specific to the research question, this

chapter defines key AVIP assessment criteria to include financial costs, opportunity

costs, risk(s) for individuals, risk(s) for force health protection, financial benefit(s) for

individuals, financial benefit(s) for force health protection, health benefit(s) for

individuals, and health benefit(s) for force health protection. These assessment criteria

---

[258]Robin L. Penslar, "Office for Human Research Protections (OHRP) IRB
Guidebook," U.S. Department of Health and Human Services, http://www.hhs.gov/
ohrp/irb/irb_guidebook.htm (accessed 30 September 2010).

[259]Ibid.

form the basis of the model used for analysis of the AVIP in chapter 4. The current

chapter further describes and characterizes data sources.

Qualitative Research Method

Qualitative research focuses on understanding behaviors, attitudes, and the social

and cultural context of a research topic.[260] Qualitative research includes statistical

analysis, intuitive, and inductive analysis.[261] Strengths of this research method include a

systematic approach, inherent collection of supporting evidence, and findings that may be

applicable beyond the immediate study.[262] Limitations of qualitative research include the

potential for variable interpretations of results.[263] In contrast, quantitative research is

focused on statistical analysis and deductive reasoning.[264] Quantitative research

frequently includes linear measurements and analysis of relationships among variables.

The qualitative method is elected in the current study, in order to promote understanding

of the context surrounding the divergent opinions regarding the AVIP.

Risks and Benefits Associated with Biodefense Vaccines

Risk assessment involves both the probability of an event and the severity of the

event. For biodefense vaccines, there is considerable uncertainty about how to determine

the probability of adverse events, as well as the probability of benefit, absent defined or

---

[260]Patricia Huston and Margo Rowan, "Qualitative Studies Their Role in Medical Research," *Canadian Family Physician* 44 (November 1998): 2454.

[261]Ibid., 2453.

[262]Ibid., 2455.

[263]Ibid., 2456.

[264]Ibid.

known risks of exposure."[265] Uncertainty regarding the probability of anthrax use as a bioweapon is a known limitation of the current study.

Financial Costs

Financial costs associated with the AVIP include the direct costs of vaccine, vaccine delivery, and vaccine administration supplies. Indirect financial costs include costs associated with cold-chain management, refrigeration and monitoring, appropriately-trained personnel to administer the vaccine, and costs associated with patient education. As the DoD utilizes similar transport media, storage facilities, vaccine administration supplies, and personnel to educate patients and deliver alternative vaccines, these costs are not considered in the current analysis. The direct cost of the anthrax vaccine is estimated based on the most recent (2008) vaccine pricing data available from the Military Vaccine (MILVAX) Agency. There are currently five vaccines in the primary anthrax vaccine series, therefore the cost per individual patient is calculated based on receipt of five doses. Financial costs for population force health protection are conservatively estimated based on the number of personnel currently deployed to the Korean Peninsula and Central Command.

Opportunity Costs

Opportunity cost describes the value of an option not selected. When a decision is made in the setting of finite resources or limited options, the chosen course of action yields opportunity but also results in the loss of alternate opportunities. For the purpose

---

[265]Gregory Poland, Robert M. Jacobson, Jon Tilburt, and Kristin Nichol, ―The Social, Political, Ethical, and Economic Aspects of Biodefense Vaccines," *Vaccine* 27 (2009): D24.

of this study, opportunity cost is described in financial terms, and mirrors the financial cost associated with the anthrax vaccine series.

Risk(s) For Individuals

Risks for individual patients associated with the AVIP include physical discomfort associated with vaccination, psychological stress associated with vaccination, and the potential of adverse vaccine reactions. These risks are described and stratified based on recent primary research data.

Risk(s) For Force Health Protection

Risks for force health protection associated with the AVIP include reductions in personnel efficacy secondary to physical or psychological discomfort associated with vaccination, and adverse vaccine reactions. Population data for adverse reaction incidence rates are used to quantify this risk. Historical fears surrounding the AVIP are an additional risk to the confidence of military personnel in the AVIP. Data that support or refute these concerns are relevant to personnel and public confidence in and compliance with current and future force health protection strategies.

Financial and Health Benefit(s) For Individuals

Financial and health benefits for individuals associated with the AVIP include a marked risk reduction of anthrax disease. This risk reduction is quantified based on historical population data. Morbidity and mortality reduction in the event of anthrax exposure is a direct health benefit associated with vaccination. In this analysis, risk reduction is also expressed in financial terms with an estimate of the cost to care for a patient with anthrax disease. Pending the time of vaccination and individual immune response, disease risk reduction may be conferred beyond military service in some patients. Patients who have received several doses of the anthrax vaccine may be compensated for donation of anthrax immune globulin-containing plasma.

Financial and Health Benefit(s) For Force Health Protection

Similar to individual financial and health benefits, in the event of disease exposure, a reduction in the number of infected service members has direct financial and health benefits for the force. In the current study, this risk reduction is extrapolated from individual patient risk reduction data.

Application of Model

This thesis enumerates current risks and benefits associated with the AVIP for individual service members and force health protection. The current, known, risks and benefits associated with the AVIP are analyzed. Over time as the body of scientific knowledge changes, and anticipated exposure risks change, interpretation of the balance between risks and benefits will not remain consistent. Assessment of current data will assist in evaluation of the AVIP as a force health protection measure and will help physicians and patients communicate regarding vaccination.

Summary

This chapter introduced the methodology used to assess current risks and benefits associated with the AVIP. Specific analysis criteria are described. The strengths and limitations of the methodology are acknowledged. The following chapter presents the data analysis.

CHAPTER 4

ANALYSIS

In combination with increasing global political instability and radical fundamentalism, valid concerns over the ability to protect the civilian population against agents of bioterrorism remain widespread. - Gregory Poland, Robert Jacobson, Jon Tilburt and Kristin Nichol, Mayo Vaccine Research Group, Mayo Clinic and Foundation.

— Gregory Poland et al., ―The Social, Political, Ethical, and Economic Aspects of Biodefense Vaccines"

Introduction

As previously introduced, the primary research question is: Based on available evidence-based literature, what are the current known risks and benefits of the AVIP? This chapter analyzes the current, known risks and benefits associated with the AVIP. Assessed criteria include financial costs, opportunity costs, risk(s) for individuals, risk(s) for force health protection, financial benefit(s) for individuals, financial benefit(s) for force health protection, health benefit(s) for individuals, and health benefit(s) for force health protection.

Financial Costs

In August 2008, the cost to the DoD per dose of anthrax vaccine was $23.33 U.S. dollars.[266] For a six-dose primary series, the cost in 2008 dollars was $139.98 dollars. Using a Consumer Price Index (CPI) inflation calculator available from the U.S. Department of Labor Bureau of Labor Statistics, table 1 illustrates the buying power of

---

[266]Military Vaccine (MILVAX) Agency, ―DoD Vaccine, Skin Test, and Antibody Price List," http://www.vaccines.mil/documents/891PriceList.xls (accessed 29 December 2010).

$23.33 in 2008 dollars for each calendar year of the AVIP below.[267] The CPI inflation

calculator uses the average CPI for a given calendar year. Data generated by the

calculator simplify the interpretation of changes in prices, and allow comparison of price

index levels over time.

Table 1.   Changes in Buying Power Associated with Anthrax Vaccine in U.S. Dollars

Year	Buying Power associated per anthrax vaccine dose in USD	Buying power associated with primary anthrax series in USD
1998	17.66	105.98
1999	18.05	108.32
2000	18.66	111.96
2001	19.19	115.14
2002	19.49	116.96
2003	19.94	119.63
2004	20.47	122.81
2005	21.16	126.97
2006	21.85	131.07
2007	22.47	134.80
2008	23.33	139.98
2009	23.25	Series changed to 5 doses December 2008; cost of primary series approximated: 23.25 x 5 = 116.25
2010	23.71	Series changed to 5 doses December 2008; cost of primary series approximated: 23.71 x 5 = 118.55

Source: Created by author using data from United States Department of Labor Bureau of Labor Statistics, ―CPI Inflation Calculator," http://data.bls.gov/cgi-bin/cpicalc.pl (accessed 29 December 2010).

---

[267]United States Department of Labor Bureau of Labor Statistics, ―CPI Inflation Calculator," http://data.bls.gov/cgi-bin/cpicalc.pl (accessed 29 December 2010).

A July 2010 Congressional Research Service report found that 207,600 contractor personnel and 175,000 military personnel support operations in Iraq and Afghanistan.[268] In March 2010, of the 112,000 contractors in Afghanistan, 16,000 were U.S. citizens.[269] In March 2010, of the 95,500 contractors in Iraq, 24,719 were U.S. citizens.[270] According to the U.S. Department of State, the Presidents of the Republic of Korea and the United States agreed to cap the number of U.S. personnel in South Korea at 28,500 in 2008.[271] Adding the number of military personnel in Iraq, Afghanistan, and South Korea in addition to the U.S. citizens serving as contractors in Iraq and Afghanistan yields a total figure of 244,219. This personnel estimate of approximately 250,000 persons eligible for the anthrax vaccine does not include contract and civilian personnel serving in the Korean Peninsula, laboratory personnel who require the anthrax vaccine for protection against occupational exposure, personnel who require the vaccine secondary to unique mission sets, adult family members accompanying military personnel in Central Command or Korea, or other personnel eligible for voluntary vaccination.

With a conservative estimate of 250,000 people eligible for the anthrax vaccine secondary to area of geographic assignment, the estimated annual cost associated with the vaccine ranges tremendously. If 250,000 persons received an annual booster, the cost

---

[268]Moshe Schwartz, R40764, *Department of Defense Contractors in Iraq and Afghanistan: Background and Analysis* (Washington, DC: Congressional Research Service, 2 July 2010): Summary.

[269]Ibid., 12.

[270]Ibid., 9.

[271]Bureau of East Asian and Pacific Affairs, ―Background Note: South Korea,‖ U.S. Department of State, http://www.state.gov/r/pa/ei/bgn/2800.htm (accessed 30 December 2010).

would be approximately $5,927,500 in 2010 dollars. If 250,000 persons received a primary anthrax series of five doses, the cost would be approximately $29,637,500.

Opportunity Costs

Evaluation of the opportunity costs associated with the AVIP must consider both financial and non-financial costs. As discussed above, direct financial costs associated with the vaccine in 2010 likely range between $6 and $30 million. These estimates do not account for the indirect administration costs associated with the AVIP to include supply and logistics costs, delivery costs, education costs, administrative costs, and medical personnel costs. As similar or overlapping costs are also associated with other DoD-mandated vaccines, these costs are acknowledged but not enumerated in the current discussion.

Non-financial opportunity costs of the AVIP include loss of personnel efficacy secondary to vaccine-related adverse events, and a detriment in internal and external organizational credibility related to the AVIP. In 2003, the Anthrax Vaccine Expert Committee (AVEC) published a review of 1,841 VAERS reports describing 3,991 adverse event reports submitted to VAERS between 1998 and 2001.[272] During this interval, more than 500,000 US military personnel received two million doses of the anthrax vaccine.[273] Reported adverse events were then summarized for demographic

---

[272] John L. Sever et al., "Safety of Anthrax Vaccine: An Expanded Review and Evaluation of Adverse Events Reported to the Vaccine Adverse Event Reporting System (VAERS)," *Pharmacoepidemiology and Drug Safety* (2004): 2.

[273] Ibid.

variables, type of event, severity, concomitant illness, and receipt of other vaccine(s).[274] One hundred forty-seven VAERS reports described a severe or medically important adverse event.[275] After a detailed case review, 26 of these 147 adverse events were characterized as having a possible, probable, or certain relationship to the vaccination.[276] Twelve of these 26 events were injection site reactions requiring brief hospitalizations, five were anaphylactic-like reactions occurred without any incidence of true anaphylaxis, and eight included a variety of other systemic reactions.[277]

Despite the low incidence of adverse events reported by the AVEC, a study of service members surveyed between 1998 and 2000 demonstrated that service members questioned the ethics, safety, and efficacy of the AVIP.[278] Multiple public and popular media sources raised concerns about the association between the anthrax vaccine and a wide range of medical conditions. Distrust of the AVIP among military members and the public prompted congressional intervention, review of the vaccine by the National Academy of Sciences in 2002, and multiple post marketing safety studies.[279]

---

[274]Ibid.

[275]Ibid.

[276]Ibid., 5.

[277]Ibid., 14.

[278]Denise Pica-Branco and Ronald P. Hudak, ―U.S. Military Service Members‘ Perceptions of the Anthrax Vaccine Immunization Program,‖ *Military Medicine* 173, no. 5 (May 2008): 429.

[279]John D. Grabenstein et al., ―Immunization to Protect the US Armed Forces: Heritage, Current Practice, and Prospects,‖ *Epidemiologic Reviews* 28 (2006): 14.

Widespread concerns regarding the anthrax vaccine has had both direct and indirect opportunity costs for the military. In addition to mistrust, and increased medical resource utilization within the military, many service members have cited the anthrax immunization program as their reason for leaving the military.[280] Concerns regarding the anthrax vaccine were not limited to military personnel. A study published in 2008 regarding the perceptions of postal workers and public health professionals following the 2001 anthrax attacks in the United States correlates with the significant public concerns regarding the anthrax vaccine in 2001.[281] Dr. Sandra Crouse Quinn, Associate Professor at the Graduate School of Public Health, University of Pittsburgh, Behavioral and Community Health Sciences et al. used data from interviews and focus groups with 65 postal workers and structured interviews with 16 public health professionals to illustrate the population's concerns.[282]

> Some postal workers reacted with suspicion to the vaccine offer, believing that they were the subjects of research, and some African American workers specifically drew an analogy to the Tuskegee syphilis study. The consent forms required for the protocol heightened mistrust. Postal workers also had complex and ambivalent responses to additional research on their health.[283]

---

[280]Committee to Assess the Safety and Efficacy of the Anthrax Vaccine and Medical Follow-Up Agency: 85; United States General Accounting Office, GAO-01-92T, *Anthrax Vaccine Preliminary Results of GAO's Survey of Guard/Reserve Pilots and Aircrew Members.*

[281]Sandra Crouse Quinn, Tammy Thomas, and Supriya Kumar, ―The Anthrax Vaccine and Research: Reactions from Postal Workers and Public Health Professionals," *Biosecurity and Bioterrorism: Biodefense Strategy, Practice, and Science* 6, no. 4 (2008): 321.

[282]Ibid.

[283]Ibid.

Quinn et al. describe a lack of trust, variability in risk perception, disagreement about treatment recommendations, and controversy over the military's use of the anthrax vaccine as factors that influenced the responses and choices of postal workers.[284]

Recognition of these costs prompted innovations in the DoD's immunization programming. According to Dr. John Grabenstein, a pharmaco-epidemiologist, and retired director of the Military Vaccine Agency, et al., public health concerns surrounding the AVIP ―pointed out needed improvements in the way the Department of Defense exchanges information with military personnel and their families and provides clinical immunization services in general."[285] In the early 2000s, the DoD initiated improved education and communication strategies to promote increased understanding of the AVIP. In 2001, the DoD and the CDC established the Vaccine Healthcare Centers Network (VHC) to ensure quality vaccine administration and improve surveillance and reporting of vaccine-associated adverse reactions in the military.[286] Currently, all vaccinees receive a current vaccine information sheet, a DoD-specific information trifold, and are encouraged to ask questions prior to the vaccine administration.

---

[284]Ibid.

[285]Grabenstein et al., 15.

[286]Vaccine Healthcare Centers Network, ―About the Vaccine Healthcare Centers Network (VHC)," http://www.vhcinfo.org/aboutUs.asp?page=about&title= AboutUs&subnav=about (accessed 3 January 2011).

Risk(s) for Individuals

Similar to other vaccines, the anthrax vaccine may cause irritation, redness, itching, swelling, and tenderness at the injection site. [287] Approximately 30 percent of men and 60 percent of women vaccines report temporary, local injection site reactions. [288] When the vaccine is given via the intramuscular versus subcutaneous route, local injection site reactions are diminished. [289] Vaccine experts speculate that this difference in local reactions may be secondary to the aluminum hydroxide adjuvant used in the anthrax vaccine. [290]

One to five percent of patients reported reactions of one to five inches in diameter. [291] Larger local reactions occurred in approximately one in 100 vaccinated patients. [292] Five to 35 percent of patients experienced systemic reactions to include muscle aches, joint pain, headaches, rash, chills, fever, nausea, loss of appetite, or malaise. [293] Allergic reactions to the anthrax vaccine have occurred less frequently than one in 100,000 doses. [294] Severe adverse reactions requiring hospitalization have occurred

---

[287] Military Vaccine (MILVAX) Agency, ―AVIP Questions and Answers,‖ http://www.anthrax. osd.mil/resource/qna/qaAll.asp?cID=309 (accessed 2 January 2011).

[288] Ibid.

[289] Emergent BioSolutions, ―BioThrax® (Anthrax Vaccine Adsorbed).‖

[290] Grabenstein et al., 15.

[291] Military Vaccine (MILVAX) Agency, ―AVIP Questions and Answers.‖

[292] Ibid.

[293] Ibid.

[294] Ibid.

approximately one in 200,000 doses.[295] In the recent 2002-2008 CDC study associated with the anthrax immunization dose and route change, of 1,564 healthy volunteers, less than one percent of patients experienced a severe adverse reaction.[296]

Historical speculation regarding associations between anthrax immunization and multiple diseases and long-term disability has increased concern regarding the vaccine. Diseases questioned as possibly associated with anthrax immunization have included systemic lupus erythematosus, hypothyroidism, diabetes, cancers, Guillain-Barre´ syndrome, and multiple sclerosis.[297] Epidemiologists have conducted objective comparisons of anthrax-immunized and anthrax-unimmunized personnel for each major diagnostic group.[298] No discrepancies were noted among the immunized and non-immunized cohorts with respect to these diseases.[299] According to Grabenstein et al., ―Several of the cohort studies span observation for multiple years after immunization. Many of the individual concerns can now be understood as instances of the post hoc ergo propter hoc fallacy.‖[300]

---

[295]Military Vaccine (MILVAX) Agency, ―AVIP Questions and Answers.‖

[296]Emergent BioSolutions, ―BioThrax® (Anthrax Vaccine Adsorbed).‖

[297]Grabenstein et al., 14-15.

[298]Ibid.

[299]Ibid.

[300]Ibid.

A study published in 1974 followed a cohort of intensively immunized laboratory personnel at Ft. Detrick over approximately 25 years.[301] Secondary to occupational risk, patients received repeated inoculations with a variety of vaccines and toxoids to include anthrax.[302] Patients had detailed medical examinations in 1956, 1962, and 1971.[303] A control group of 26 age- and gender-matched, civilian employees from Fort Detrick, who had never received special immunizations and had never been exposed to laboratory infections was additionally studied.[304] No clinical illnesses attributable to long-term immunizations were identified in the study group.[305]

Risk(s) For Force Health Protection

Risks for the force associated with the AVIP include lost productivity secondary to physical or psychological discomfort associated with vaccination, and adverse vaccine reactions. Although severe adverse reactions to the AVIP are rare as detailed above, severe adverse events affect medical readiness, and force efficacy. Historical fears surrounding the AVIP are an additional risk to the confidence of military personnel in the AVIP. Data that support or refute these concerns are relevant to personnel and public confidence in and compliance with current and future force health protection strategies.

---

[301]Charles S. White, III, William H. Adler, and Virginia G. McGann, "Repeated Immunization: Possible Adverse Effects Reevaluation of Human Subjects at 25 Years," *Annals of Internal Medicine* 81 (1974): 594.

[302]Ibid.

[303]Ibid.

[304]Ibid., 595.

[305]Ibid., 594.

<u>Financial and Health Benefit(s) For Individuals</u>
<u>and Force Health Protection</u>

The 2002 Institute of Medicine review of AVA safety and efficacy data concluded

that the AVA demonstrates effective vaccine protection of humans.[306] Further, the

committee determined that AVA's mechanism protects humans from multiple *B.*

anthracis strains and that a novel natural bioengineered strain would probably not

overcome the vaccine.[307]

The 2009 ACIP Recommendations for the Use of Anthrax Vaccine in the United

States specifically addressed the potential benefit of pre-exposure anthrax vaccination.

> By priming the immune system before exposure to *B. anthracis* spores, pre-event
> and preexposure vaccination might provide more protection than antimicrobial
> agents alone to persons at risk for occupational exposure to *B. anthracis,*
> including protection for persons exposed to large inocula, protection if the public
> health infrastructure cannot ensure immediate availability or timely delivery of
> postevent antimicrobial agents, and potential benefits if bioengineered strains
> were released, limiting antimicrobial PEP effectiveness.[308]

Limitations in health infrastructure, risk of large inocula, and risk of exposure to

bioengineered strains of *B. anthracis* are relevant concerns for service members and force

health protection.

In a 2005 study, Dr. Robert Fowler of the Sunnybrook and Women's College

Health Sciences Centre, University of Toronto, et al. compared the cost-effectiveness of

---

[306]Advisory Committee on Immunization Practices. ―Use of Anthrax Vaccine in
the United States Recommendations of the Advisory Committee on Immunization
Practices (ACIP), 2009," 10.

[307]Ibid.

[308]Ibid., 19.

vaccination and antibiotic prophylaxis against anthrax infection.[309] The study modeled a

civilian rather than military population, and compared outcomes associated with pre-

attack and post-attack anthrax prevention and treatment strategies.[310] Although the study

does not directly address a military population, the findings yield relevant data that may

be applicable to various populations. According to Fowler et al., costs associated with a

perceived or real anthrax bioterrorism incident are estimated at more than $26 billion per

100,000 people.[311] Using 2004 US dollars, Fowler et al. estimated the inpatient costs

associated with moderate inhalational anthrax at $5,361 per person per day, and the

inpatient costs associated with severe inhalational anthrax at $28,731 per person per

day.[312] Estimated oral antibiotic costs range from $12 to $3,600 per day for 60 days.[313]

The authors concluded that post-exposure vaccines plus antibiotics for post-

exposure anthrax prophylaxis were the most effective strategy in their model.[314]

However, they acknowledged the mechanism of anthrax release and exposure estimates

as limitations: ―Our most important finding about pre-attack vaccination is that the net

---

[309]Robert A. Fowler et al., ―Cost-Effectiveness of Defending Against Bioterrorism: A Comparison of Vaccination and Antibiotic Prophylaxis Against Anthrax,‖ *Annals of Internal Medicine* 142, no. 8 (19 April 2005): 601.

[310]Ibid., 602.

[311]Ibid., 601.

[312]Ibid., 604.

[313]Ibid.

[314]Ibid., 607.

health benefit and cost-effectiveness depended critically on the probability of an attack and on the proportion of the population exposed during the attack."[315]

The authors concluded that a pre-exposure vaccination provides a net cost and quality of life benefit at "relatively low probabilities" of clinically significant anthrax exposure (1 in 500).[316] This transition to benefit associated with pre-exposure vaccination at a low exposure risk has obvious implications for the military. Additionally, the Fowler et al. model relies on seamless, rapid delivery of post-exposure antibiotics and vaccine to make sole reliance on post-exposure vaccine and antibiotic prophylaxis the most effective strategy. "Our results suggest that if distribution of antibiotics or adherence to antibiotics is substantially impaired, previous vaccination may become cost-effective."[317] This "finding is consistent with the work of other authors who have estimated greater than 50 percent increases in post-attack mortality rate when either the distribution of antibiotics is delayed or prophylactic adherence to antibiotics is substantially diminished."[318] In austere civilian and military settings, both medication delivery and adherence must be questioned.

In 2007, Dr. Brian Schmitt of the Medicine and Neurology Service Line and Department of Medicine, Hines VA Medical Center, Hines, Ill, and Stritch School of Medicine, Loyola University Chicago, et al. conducted a cost-effectiveness analysis comparing pre-attack vaccination with post-attack antibiotic treatment and vaccination in

---

[315]Ibid., 607-608.

[316]Ibid., 608.

[317]Ibid.

[318]Ibid.

a hypothetical small-scale anthrax bioterrorism incident in a US Postal Service distribution center in a large metropolitan center.[319] Schmitt et al. based treatment and cost assumptions on the anthrax cases from the 2001 postal attacks. In the Schmitt et al. model, inhalational anthrax survivors were hospitalized for 14 days, received intravenous antibiotics for seven days, received oral antibiotics for 53 days, and received biannual follow-up visits following recovery.[320] Patients who died from inhalational anthrax were hospitalized for three days.[321] Treatment for patients with inhalational anthrax who survived was estimated in 2005 dollars at $26,343.34.[322] Treatment for patients with inhalational anthrax who did not survive was estimated in 2005 dollars at $5,493.50.[323] Schmitt et al. concluded that in a small-scale attack, post-attack antibiotic therapy and vaccination of exposed personnel is the preferred strategy because of assumed low exposure risk, infectious dose, and anticipated high therapy adherence.[324] These constraints are not present in large-scale attacks.

Fowler et al. and Schmitt et al. both estimate financial costs associated with vaccine-related and antibiotic-related adverse events. Both studies suggested that similar

[319]Brian Schmitt et al., ─Responding to a Small-scale Bioterrorist Anthrax Attack: Cost-effectiveness Analysis Comparing Preattack Vaccination With Postattack Antibiotic Treatment and Vaccination," *Archives of Internal Medicine* 167, no. 7 (9 April 2007): 655.

[320]Ibid., 657.

[321]Ibid.

[322]Ibid., 656.

[323]Ibid.

[324]Ibid., 661.

costs are associated with vaccine-related adverse events and antibiotic-related adverse events. Schmitt et al. provided the same estimate for the cost of a mild adverse reaction to anthrax vaccine and the cost of a mild adverse reaction to antibiotics: $89.64 in 2005 US dollars.[325] Schmitt et al. also provided the same estimate for the cost of a severe adverse reaction to anthrax vaccine and the cost of a severe adverse reaction to antibiotics: $3,841.62 in 2005 dollars.[326] Fowler et al. provided similar estimates for the financial costs associated with adverse reactions. Fowler et al. estimated the cost of mild, moderate, and severe vaccine-related adverse events at $8, $18, and $2,473 respectively in 2004 US dollars.[327] Fowler et al. estimated the costs of mild, moderate, and severe antibiotic-related adverse events at $10, $103, and $2,473 respectively in 2004 dollars.[328] The relative parity in costs associated with adverse events suggests that the risk of post-exposure antibiotics in both models may be similar to the risk of vaccination.

Summary

This chapter reviews recent and current scientific data regarding the known risks and benefits associated with the AVIP. The direct and indirect financial costs associated with the anthrax vaccine are significant. From a force management perspective, financial costs associated with the anthrax vaccine may impact spending in alternate areas. The anthrax vaccine is associated with local adverse reactions in approximately 30-60 percent

---

[325]Ibid., 656.

[326]Ibid.

[327]Fowler et al., 604.

[328]Ibid.

of patients. However, prior studies have demonstrated that less than one percent of patients experience a severe adverse reaction. Historical fears surrounding anthrax vaccine association with systemic disease have been disproven by ongoing scientific study. Independent evaluations of the anthrax vaccine by civilian organizations to include the Institute of Medicine and the ACIP have yielded reassuring results, and have suggested that the anthrax vaccine may be the most efficacious prevention strategy for patients with high exposure risk and impaired access to post-exposure treatment. Additional civilian-sponsored risk modeling analyses have demonstrated the astounding costs and mortality associated with inhalational anthrax exposure. Interestingly, similar costs are estimated for vaccine-related adverse events and antibiotic-related adverse events.

Limitations of the analysis, specifically the ability to apply all civilian-sponsored research to the unique population and unique risks of service members, are acknowledged. The following chapter presents the conclusions and recommendations for future study.

CHAPTER 5

CONCLUSIONS AND RECOMMENDATIONS

The AVIP protects service members against a potent, invisible, and intangible threat. Offensive and defensive biological weapons programs throughout the world have studied anthrax for most of the last century. Domestic and international organizations to include the United States Department of Homeland Security, the DoD, the CDC, and the WHO have all explicitly recognized anthrax as a bioterrorism threat.[329] The accidental release of anthrax in 1979 in the former Soviet Union, and the 2001 bioterrorism incident in the United States leave little disagreement about the human health threat associated with inhalation anthrax exposure. Based on available evidence-based literature, the AVIP has both risks and benefits for the force and for individual service members. Although the risk of anthrax exposure is difficult to quantify, the benefits associated with vaccine protection outweigh the risks associated with vaccination.

Lessons Learned from Civilian Response

Despite long-standing recognition of anthrax as a bioterrorism threat, the 2001 intentional release of anthrax spores in the United States resulted in five fatalities among the 11 documented cases of inhalation anthrax.[330] In the subsequent decade, federal organizations have studied and instituted several initiatives to decrease the public health

---

[329]Advisory Committee on Immunization Practices, ―Use of Anthrax Vaccine in the United States Recommendations of the Advisory Committee on Immunization Practices (ACIP), 2009,‖ 3-4.

[330]Mark B. Stephens and Blake Marvin, ―Recognition of Community-Acquired Anthrax: Has Anything Changed Since 2001?‖ *Military Medicine* 175, no. 9 (September 2010): 671.

risk associated with anthrax. An October 2003 General Accounting Office report on the

public health system response to the 2001 anthrax attacks reported on both strengths and

deficiencies in the public health system's response. Public health officials reported that

elements of public health response systems to include laboratories, timely clinical

guidelines, and effective communication were severely strained.[331] Public health officials

speculated that if the incidents had been prolonged or more extensive, response would

have been difficult to sustain.[332]

Limitations in the relatively resource-rich public health response to the 2001

anthrax release may portend greater potential limitations in austere military settings.

Although logistics, communication, and patient adherence to prescribed medication

regimens may be significant strengths of military medicine in the non-combat setting,

deployed military settings may involve large distances, poor communication, and

increased transition time between levels of care. A large-scale debilitating illness within a

vulnerable population could severely strain the medical and logistic capabilities of a

deployed force.

Conclusions

Aggregate data from long-term studies and review by multiple scientific

organizations, both within and external to the DoD, suggest that the AVA is both safe and

efficacious. Animal studies, a controlled vaccine trial in humans, human observational

---

[331]United States General Accounting Office, GAO-04-152, *Bioterrorism: Public Health Response to Anthrax Incidents of 2001* (Washington, DC: Government Printing Office, October 2003), 4.

[332]Ibid.

data, and human and other mammal immunogenicity data are the basis for AVA efficacy data.[333] Specific vaccine efficacy conclusions regarding inhalational anthrax are drawn from challenges of Rhesus macaques and observational human data from mill workers between 1955 and 1959.[334] Vaccine safety data are based on both pre-licensure and extensive post-licensure studies. Service members have represented the majority of vaccine recipients since inception of the AVIP. Between January 1998 and December 2008, approximately 12.4 million doses of anthrax vaccine were distributed by the manufacturer for DoD and domestic licensed use.[335] The military received more than 99 percent of this vaccine distribution.[336] Between March 1998 and December 2008, approximately 8.4 million doses were administered to approximately 2.1 million military personnel.[337]

Patients do experience known adverse reactions in association with AVA. Approximately 30 percent of men and 60 percent of women report temporary, local injection site reactions.[338] One to five percent of patients report local reactions of one to five inches in diameter.[339] However, less than one percent of patients experience a severe

---

[333]Advisory Committee on Immunization Practices. ―Use of Anthrax Vaccine in the United States Recommendations of the Advisory Committee on Immunization Practices (ACIP), 2009," 9.

[334]Ibid., 9-10.

[335]Ibid., 11.

[336]Ibid.

[337]Ibid.

[338]Military Vaccine (MILVAX) Agency, ―AVIP Questions and Answers."

[339]Ibid.

adverse reaction.[340] These adverse reaction rates are not markedly divergent from adverse reaction rates associated with other vaccines. According to the CDC, in placebo-controlled studies of the trivalent inactivated influenza vaccine (―flu shot") in adults, 10-64 percent of patients reported soreness at the site of vaccination that lasted less than two days.[341] The rate of serious adverse events among adults following the trivalent inactivated influenza vaccine was less than one percent.[342]

A gender discrepancy with more adverse events reported in women, is also reported in association with both childhood and adult vaccines to include the Influenza, Yellow Fever, Measles, Mumps, and Rubella, and Japanese Encephalitis Virus vaccines.[343] This discrepancy among adverse event symptoms between genders is not fully understood.[344] Different inflammatory and cellular immune responses among genders may affect viral clearance and disease symptoms.[345] Variations in immune responses among genders vaccines may explain differences in adverse event rates in association with vaccines.[346] Alternatively, a reporting bias among the genders, with

---

[340]Emergent BioSolutions, ―BioThrax® (Anthrax Vaccine Adsorbed)."

[341]Centers for Disease Control and Prevention, ―2010-11 Influenza Prevention," http://www.cdc.gov/flu/professionals/acip/adverseTIV.htm (accessed 11 February 2011).

[342]Ibid.

[343]Sabra L. Klein, Anne Jedlicka, and Andrew Pekosz, ―The Xs and Y of Immune Responses to Viral Vaccines," *The Lancet Infectious Diseases* 10 (May 2010): 339.

[344]Ibid., 338.

[345]Ibid.

[346]Ibid.

higher adverse reporting rates among women, may also explain this discrepancy in adverse event rates.[347]

AVA is the only licensed anthrax vaccine in the United States. Currently, there is no alternative pre-exposure prophylactic vaccine. In 2002, the CDC cautiously provided interim guidance for the use of antibiotics and personal protective equipment for decontamination workers responding to intentional distribution of anthrax.[348] According to the CDC, ―Despite appropriate PPE and procedures, however, there will remain a potential for breaches of protection and contamination of the workers.‖[349] However, in the event of known exposure to aerosolized anthrax, both the ACIP and the Johns Hopkins Working Group on Civilian Biodefense recommended prolonged antibiotic therapy in conjunction with anthrax vaccination as the best disease prevention strategy.[350] Based on limited animal studies, the 2002 Institute of Medicine Report on anthrax vaccine safety and efficacy also concluded that vaccine in conjunction with antibiotics following exposure may help to prevent inhalation anthrax.[351]

---

[347]Ibid.

[348]Centers for Disease Control and Prevention, ―Antimicrobial Prophylaxis to Prevent Anthrax Among Decontamination/Cleanup Workers Responding to an Intentional Distribution of Bacillus Anthracis,‖ http://emergency.cdc.gov/agent/ anthrax/exposure/cleanupprophylaxis.asp (accessed 11 February 2011).

[349]Ibid.

[350]Ibid.

[351]Ibid.

Recommendations for Policy

The DoD has tailored current AVIP policy to protect forces with anticipated high exposure risk. In addition to patients with anticipated occupational exposure, current policy mandates anthrax vaccination for service members, emergency essential civilian employees and contractors geographically deployed to Central Command or Korea areas of responsibility for 15 or more consecutive days. These geographic recommendations consider the preponderance of countries known or suspected to have bioweapons programs. Tailoring vaccination policy to anticipated risk minimizes vaccine-associated risk for individuals and for the force.

Current AVIP benefits for individuals and for force protection outweigh the limited risks for individuals and force protection. As risks and benefits change over time, ongoing assessment is essential to ensure that individual and force health promotion are optimized. The DoD has improved patient education, risk communication, and documentation related to anthrax vaccination within the past decade. Continuing long-term scientific safety and efficacy research, ongoing educational efforts, and recognition of patient concerns are essential for the continued success of the AVIP and other force protection programs. It is very reasonable for a well patient to question an intervention that involves known risk and abstract benefit. Candid presentation of the facts and fallacies of both risk and benefit are essential.

Recommendations for Future Study

Ongoing anthrax vaccine research is currently underway. In September 2010, the Biomedical Advanced Research and Development Authority (BARDA) of the DHHS awarded Emergent BioSolutions a contract for the development of a recombinant protective antigen (rPA) anthrax vaccine.[352] The recombinant protective antigen vaccine candidate is a purified recombinant protective antigen protein formulated with an adjuvant, designed to induce antibodies.[353] This vaccine candidate is based on work from the USAMRIID and has been studied previously by the National Institute of Allergy and Infectious Diseases (NIAID).[354] The candidate vaccine is desirable because it may provide enhanced immune response with fewer vaccine doses. Ongoing research into improved vaccine safety and efficacy to include novel vaccines will benefit both individual service members and force protection efforts.

A 2010 study on physicians' ability to recognize the presentation of anthrax disease underscores the need for vigilant force protection, to include focused educational programming for the civilian and military medical communities.[355] A sample of randomly selected military and civilian family physicians completed a voluntary survey based on three case vignettes adapted from the 2001 inhalational anthrax cases.[356] Participants were asked to list differential diagnoses and initial management and treatment plans.[357]

---

[352]Emergent BioSolutions Inc., ―Emergent BioSolutions Awarded HHS Contract Valued at up to $186.6 Million to Develop rPA Anthrax Vaccine," http://investors.emergentbiosolutions.com/phoenix.zhtml?c=202582&p=irol-newsArticle&ID=1472596&highlight= (accessed 11 February 2011).

[353]Ibid.

[354]Ibid.

[355]Stephens and Marvin, 671.

[356]Ibid.

[357]Ibid.

One hundred sixty four physicians completed the survey.[358] Fifty two percent of the respondents were military physicians, 68 percent had completed their residency training prior to 2001, and 59 percent were from the East Coast of the United States.[359] The most common diagnosis responses by respondents were influenza and pneumonia.[360] Only six respondents included inhalational anthrax as a diagnostic possibility on any case.[361] The authors found that differential diagnoses and clinical decision-making did not differ between military and civilian physicians, and concluded that inhalational anthrax is not frequently considered by community-based primary care physicians when confronted with an acute case of respiratory illness.[362] This finding emphasizes the need for ongoing education for both international and domestic disaster and bioterrorism response.

The military has several unique resources that could provide expert guidance and assistance in the event of a future bioterrorism event within the United States. These resources include scientific experts in anthrax biodefense, extensive research data on the AVIP within the military population, an anthrax-immunized population, and physicians experienced in AVA delivery and management. Further study and coordination are critical to ensure that this base of knowledge and resources can be mobilized to benefit both military personnel and civilians in the event of future crisis.

---

[358]Ibid., 672.

[359]Ibid.

[360]Ibid., 671.

[361]Ibid., 674.

[362]Ibid.

Anthrax is considered one of the most likely biological warfare agents. Anthrax is highly lethal, stable, and readily weaponized. Multiple countries that are hostile to the United States are known or suspected to possess anthrax. Historical fears surrounding the vaccine complicated implementation of the AVIP in the late 1990s and early 2000s. Recent studies have added additional evidence-based information about AVA safety and efficacy to the scientific literature. Although no vaccine is entirely risk-free, the benefits of protection against anthrax for both individual patients and the force far outweigh the current, known risks associated with anthrax vaccination.

GLOSSARY

Adverse Event. Any undesirable and unintended occurrence noted in association with the administration of a vaccine. An adverse event is not necessarily caused by the vaccine. Adverse events may range from mild to severe.

Anthrax Vaccine Adsorbed (AVA). A vaccine used to promote increased resistance to *B. anthracis* by active immunization.

Anthrax Vaccine Immunization Program (AVIP). The Department of Defense Anthrax Vaccine Immunization Program. Prior to December 2008, the primary anthrax vaccination series included six immunizations. Since December 2008, the primary anthrax vaccine series has included five immunizations over an 18 month period. Service members with ongoing geographic or occupational risk factors receive subsequent annual boosters.

Benefit. A desired or advantageous outcome.

Risk. The probability of harm in association with an intervention. Risk may include physical, psychological, social, or economic harm; or a combination.

BIBLIOGRAPHY

Books

Committee to Assess the Safety and Efficacy of the Anthrax Vaccine, Medical Follow-
Up Agency. *The Anthrax Vaccine: Is It Safe? Does It Work?* Washington, DC:
National Academies Press, 2002.

Darling, Robert G., and Jon B. Woods., ed. *USAMRIID's Medical Management of
Biological Casualties Handbook.* 5th ed. Frederick, MD: U.S. Army Medical
Research Institute of Infectious Diseases, 1994.

Turnbull, P. C. B. ―Guidelines for the Surveillance and Control of Anthrax in Human and
Animals. 3rd ed." *World Health Organization Emerging and other
Communicable Diseases, Surveillance and Control WHO/EMC/ZDI/98.6.*
http://www.who.int/csr/resources/publications/anthrax/whoemczdi986text.pdf
(accessed 18 October 2010).

Periodicals

Advisory Committee on Immunization Practices. ―Notice to Readers: Use of Anthrax
Vaccine in Response to Terrorism: Supplemental Recommendations of the
Advisory Committee on Immunization Practices." *MMWR Recommendations and
Reports* 51, no. 45 (15 November 2002): 1024-26.

———. ―Use of Anthrax Vaccine in the United States." *MMWR Recommendations and
Reports* 49 (15 December 2000): 1-20.

———. ―Use of Anthrax Vaccine in the United States Recommendations of the Advisory
Committee on Immunization Practices (ACIP), 2009." *MMWR Recommendations
and Reports* 59, no. RR-6 (23 July 2010): 1-30.

Bales, Michael, Andrew L. Dannenberg, Philip S. Brachman, Arnold F. Kaufmann, Peter
C. Klatsky, and David A. Ashford. ―Epidemiologic Response to Anthrax
Outbreaks: Field Investigations, 1950-2001." *Emerging Infectious Diseases* 8, no.
9 (2002): 1163-74.

Centers for Disease Control and Prevention. ―Surveillance for Adverse Events Associated
with Anthrax Vaccination-U.S. Department of Defense, 1998–2000." *MMWR
Recommendations and Reports* 49, no 16 (28 April 2000): 341-5.

———. ―Update: Investigation of Bioterrorism-Related Anthrax and Interim Guidelines
for Clinical Evaluation of Persons with Possible Anthrax." *Morbidity and
Mortality Weekly Report* 50, no. 43 (2 November 2001): 941-48.

Cieslak, Theodore, J., and Edward M. Eitzen Jr. "Clinical and Epidemiologic Principles of Anthrax." *Emerging Infectious Diseases* 5, no. 4 (July-August 1999): 552-55.

Davis, Jim, and Anna Johnson-Winegar. "The Anthrax Terror DoD's Number-One Biological Threat." *Aerospace Power Journal* (Winter 2000): 15-29.

Fowler, Robert A., Gillian D. Sanders, Dena M. Bravata, Bahman Nouri, Jason M. Gastwirth, Dane Peterson, Allison G. Broker, Alan M. Garber, and Douglas K. Owens. "Cost-Effectiveness of Defending Against Bioterrorism: A Comparison of Vaccination and Antibiotic Prophylaxis Against Anthrax." *Annals of Internal Medicine* 142, no. 8 (19 April 2005): 601-11.

Grabenstein, John D. "Countering Anthrax: Vaccines and Immunoglobulins." *Clinical Infectious Diseases* 45 (15 December 2007): 129-36.

Grabenstein, John D., Phillip R. Pittman, John T. Greenwood, and Renata J. M. Engler. "Immunization to Protect the US Armed Forces: Heritage, Current Practice, and Prospects." *Epidemiologic Reviews* 28 (2006): 3-26.

Huston, Patricia, and Margo Rowan. "Qualitative Studies Their Role in Medical Research." *Canadian Family Physician* 44 (November 1998): 2453-58.

Jernigan, Daniel, B. Pratima, L. Raghunathan, Beth P. Bell, Ross Brechner, Eddy A. Bresnitz, Jay C. Butler, Marty Cetron, Mitch Cohen, Timothy Doyle, Marc Fischer, Carolyn Greene, Kevin S. Griffith, Jeannette Guarner, James L. Hadler, James A. Hayslett, Richard Meyer, Lyle R. Petersen, Michael Phillips, Robert Pinner, Tanja Popovic, Conrad P. Quinn, Jennita Reefhuis, Dori Reissman, Nancy Rosenstein, Anne Schuchat, Wun-Ju Shieh, Larry Siegal, David L. Swerdlow, Fred C. Tenover, Marc Traeger, John W. Ward, Isaac Weisfuse, Steven Wiersma, Kevin Yeskey, Sherif Zaki, David A. Ashford, Bradley A. Perkins, Steve Ostroff, James Hughes, David Fleming, Jeffrey P. Koplan, Julie L. Gerberding, and the National Anthrax Epidemiologic Investigation Team. "Investigation of Bioterrorism-Related Anthrax, United States, 2001: Epidemiologic Findings." *Emerging Infectious Diseases* 8, no. 10 (2002): 1019-28.

LaForce, F. Marc. "Anthrax." *Clinical Infectious Diseases* 19 (December 1994): 1009-14.

Klein, Sabra L., Anne Jedlicka, and Andrew Pekosz. "The Xs and Ys of Immune Responses to Viral Vaccines." *The Lancet Infectious Diseases* 10 (May 2010): 338-49.

Nass, Meryl. "The Anthrax Vaccine Program: An Analysis of the CDC's Recommendations for Vaccine Use." *American Journal of Public Health* 92, no. 5 (May 2002): 715-21.

Pica-Branco, Denise, and Ronald P. Hudak. "U.S. Military Service Members' Perceptions of the Anthrax Vaccine Immunization Program." *Military Medicine* 173, no. 5 (May 2008): 429-33.

Poland, Gregory, Robert M. Jacobson, Jon Tilburt, and Kristin Nichol. "The Social, Political, Ethical, and Economic Aspects of Biodefense Vaccines." *Vaccine* 27 (2009): D23-D27.

Quinn, Sandra Crouse, Tammy Thomas, and Supriya Kumar. "The Anthrax Vaccine and Research: Reactions from Postal Workers and Public Health Professionals." *Biosecurity and Bioterrorism: Biodefense Strategy, Practice, and Science* 6, no. 4 (2008): 321-33.

Rempfer, Thomas L. "The Anthrax Vaccine: A Dilemma for Homeland Security." *Homeland Security Affairs* 5, no. 2 (May 2009): 1-12.

Ryan, Margaret A. K., Tyler C. Smith, Carter J. Sevick, William K. Honner, Rosha A. Loach, Cynthia A. Moore, and J. David Erickson. "Birth Defects Among Infants Born to Women Who Received Anthrax Vaccine In Pregnancy." *American Journal of Epidemiology* 168, no. 4 (2 July 2008): 434-42.

Schmitt, Brian, Deborah Dobrez, Jorge P. Parada, Demetrios N. Kyriacou, Robert M. Golub, Rishi Sharma, and Charles Bennett. "Responding to a Small-scale Bioterrorist Anthrax Attack: Cost-effectiveness Analysis Comparing Preattack Vaccination With Postattack Antibiotic Treatment and Vaccination." *Archives of Internal Medicine* 167, no 7 (9 April 2007): 655-62.

Sever, John L., Alan I. Brenner, Arnold D. Gale, Jerry M. Lyle, Lawrence H. Moulton, Brian J. Ward, and David J. West. "Safety of Anthrax Vaccine: An Expanded Review and Evaluation of Adverse Events Reported to the Vaccine Adverse Event Reporting System (VAERS)." *Pharmacoepidemiology and Drug Safety* (2004).

Smith, Kendall A. "Wanted, an Anthrax Vaccine: Dead or Alive?" *Medical Immunology* 4, no. 5 (18 April 2005): 1-6. http://www.medimmunol.com/content/pdf/1476-9433-4-5.pdf (accessed 17 October 2010).

Stephens, Mark B., and Blake Marvin. "Recognition of Community-Acquired Anthrax: Has Anything Changed Since 2001?" *Military Medicine* 175, no. 9 (September 2010): 671-75.

Turnbull, Peter C. B. "Anthrax Vaccines: Past, Present, and Future." *Vaccine* 9 (1991): 533-539.

White, Charles S. III, William H. Adler, and Virginia G. McGann. "Repeated Immunization: Possible Adverse Effects Reevaluation of Human Subjects at 25 Years." *Annals of Internal Medicine* 81 (1974): 594-600.

Wiesen, Andrew R., and Christopher L. Littell. "Relationship Between Prepregnancy Anthrax Vaccination and Pregnancy and Birth Outcomes Among US Army Women." *Journal of the American Medical Association* 287, no. 12 (27 March 2002): 1556-60.

Zoon, Kathryn C. "Vaccines, Pharmaceutical Products, and Bioterrorism: Challenges for the U.S. Food and Drug Administration." *Emerging Infectious Diseases* 5, no. 4 (July-August 1999): 534-36.

Government Documents

Assistant Secretary of Defense. *Continuation of the Anthrax Vaccine Immunization Program (AVIP)*. Memorandum. Washington, DC: Department of Defense, 22 December 2005.

Bureau of East Asian and Pacific Affairs. "Background Note: South Korea." Department of State. http://www.state.gov/r/pa/ei/bgn/2800.htm (accessed 30 December 2010).

Centers for Disease Control and Prevention. National Center for Zoonotic, Vector-Borne, and Enteric Diseases. "Anthrax." http://www.cdc.gov/nczved/divisions/ dfbmd/diseases/anthrax/#how_common (accessed 10 September 2010).

Department of the Army. *Temporarily Stop Giving Anthrax Immunizations to All DOD Personnel*. Memorandum. Washington, DC: Department of the Army, 24 December 2003.

Department of Defense. "What You Need to Know about Anthrax Vaccine." http://www.anthrax.mil/documents/1106AvipTrifold.pdf (accessed 4 November 2010).

Department of Health And Human Services. Food and Drug Administration. "Biological Products; Bacterial Vaccines and Toxoids; Implementation of Efficacy Review; Anthrax Vaccine Adsorbed; Final Rule and Final Order." *Federal Register* 70, no. 242 (19 December 2005), 75180-98. http://www.fda.gov/ohrms/dockets/98fr/05-24223.pdf (accessed 15 September 2010).

Deputy Secretary of Defense. *Additional Temporary Slowing and Future Resumption of Anthrax Vaccine Immunization Program (AVIP)*. Memorandum. Washington, DC: Deputy Secretary of Defense, 27 November 2000.

———. *Anthrax Vaccine Immunization Program (AVIP)*. Memorandum. Washington, DC: Deputy Secretary of Defense, 12 October 2006.

———. *Reintroduction of the Anthrax Vaccine Immunization Program (AVIP)*. Memorandum. Washington, DC: Deputy Secretary of Defense, 28 June 2002.

———. *Resumption of the Anthrax Vaccine Immunization Program (AVIP) Under Emergency Use Authorization (EUA)*. Memorandum. Washington, DC: Deputy Secretary of Defense, 25 April 2005.

———. *Temporary Slowing and Future Resumption of Anthrax Vaccine Immunization Program (AVIP)*. Memorandum. Washington, DC: Deputy Secretary of Defense, 17 July 2000.

Military Vaccine (MILVAX) Agency. Office of The Army Surgeon General. ―Anthrax Vaccine Immunization Program (AVIP) Questions and Answers." http://www.anthrax.osd.mil/documents/Anthrax_QA.pdf (accessed 23 November 2010): 1-61.

———. ―AVIP Anthrax Vaccine Immunization Program." http://www.anthrax.osd.mil/default.asp (accessed 7 November 2010).

———. ―AVIP Questions and Answers." http://www.anthrax.osd.mil/resource/qna/qaAll.asp?cID=309 (accessed 2 January 2011).

———. ―DoD Vaccine, Skin Test, and Antibody Price List." http://www.vaccines.mil/documents/891PriceList.xls (accessed 29 December 2010).

Schwartz, Moshe. R40764, *Department of Defense Contractors in Iraq and Afghanistan: Background and Analysis*. Washington, DC: Congressional Research Service, July 2010.

Secretary of the Army. *Slowdown of the Anthrax Vaccine Immunization Program (AVIP)*. Washington, DC: Secretary of the Army, 8 June 2001.

Secretary of Defense. *Anthrax Vaccine Immunization Program Pause*. Memorandum. Washington, DC: Secretary of Defense, 27 October 2004.

———. *Implementation of the Anthrax Vaccination Program for the Total Force*. Memorandum. Washington, DC: Secretary of Defense, 18 May 1998.

Under Secretary of Defense. *Anthrax Vaccine Immunization Program*. Memorandum. Washington, DC: Under Secretary of Defense, 23 December 2003.

———. *Anthrax Vaccine Immunization Program Resumption*. Memorandum. Washington, DC: Under Secretary of Defense, 7 January 2004.

———. *Change to Anthrax Vaccine Immunization Program (AVIP) Operational Procedure (One Day Policy)*. Memorandum. Washington, DC: Under Secretary of Defense, 30 March 1999.

———. *Implementation of the Anthrax Vaccine Immunization Program (AVIP)*. Memorandum. Washington, DC: Under Secretary of Defense, December 2006.

United States Department of Labor Bureau of Labor Statistics. ―CPI Inflation Calculator.‖ http://data.bls.gov/cgi-bin/cpicalc.pl (accessed 29 December 2010).

United States District Court for the District of Columbia. Civil Action No. 06-2131, *Thomas Rempfer, et al., v. Andrew C. Von Eschenbach, Commissioner Food and Drug Administration, et al.* http://www.anthrax.mil/documents/library/ AnthraxAppealDismissal.pdf (accessed 12 November 2010).

United States Food and Drug Administration. ―Review of VAERS Anthrax Vaccine Reports Received through 8/15/05, and Adverse Event Reports Submitted to Docket No. 1980N-0208.‖ 13 December 2005. http://www.anthrax.mil/ documents/965VAERSvol225.pdf (accessed 9 November 2010).

———. ―Vaccine Product Approval Process.‖ http://www.fda.gov/biologicsblood vaccines/developmentapprovalprocess/biologicslicenseapplicationsblaprocess/uc m133096.htm (accessed 11 November 2010).

———. Bioterrorism and Drug Preparedness.‖FDA Approves License Supplements For Anthrax Vaccine.‖ http://www.fda.gov/Drugs/EmergencyPreparedness/ BioterrorismandDrugPreparedness/ucm133146.htm (accessed 12 September 2010).

———. Vaccines, Blood and Biologics. ―Anthrax.‖ http://www.fda.gov/biologicsblood vaccines/vaccines/ucm061751.htm (accessed 28 October 2010).

United States General Accounting Office. GAO-01-92T, *Anthrax Vaccine Preliminary Results of GAO's Survey of Guard/Reserve Pilots and Aircrew Members.* Washington, DC: Government Printing Office, October 2000.

———. GAO-04-152, *Bioterrorism: Public Health Response to Anthrax Incidents of 2001.* Washington, DC: Government Printing Office, October 2003.

———. GAO/T-NSIAD-99-148, *Safety and Efficacy of the Anthrax Vaccine.* Washington, DC: Government Printing Office, 29 April 1999.

Other Sources

BBC News, ―Britain's _Anthrax Island',‖ 25 July 2001. http://news.bbc.co.uk/ 1/hi/scotland/1457035.stm (accessed 2 December 2010).

Centers for Disease Control and Prevention. ―2010-11 Influenza Prevention.‖ http://www.cdc.gov/flu/professionals/acip/adverseTIV.htm (accessed 11 February 2011).

———. ―Anthrax Q and A.‖ http://emergency.cdc.gov/agent/anthrax/faq/preventive.asp (accessed 11 February 2011).

———. Emergency Preparedness and Response. ―Anthrax Q and A: Preventive Therapy.‖ http://www.bt.cdc.gov/agent/anthrax/faq/ preventive.asp (accessed 19 October 2010).

———. ―Antimicrobial Prophylaxis to Prevent Anthrax among Decontamination/ CleanupWorkers Responding to an Intentional Distribution of Bacillus Anthracis.‖ http://emergency.cdc.gov/agent/anthrax/exposure/ cleanupprophylaxis.asp (accessed 11 February 2011).

The Cochrane Collaboration. ―Cochrane Reviews.‖ http://www.cochrane.org/cochrane-reviews (accessed 11 November 2010).

Curry, COL Donald G. Jr. ―The Case for ‗Forced‗ Health Protection.‖ U.S. Army War College Strategy Research Project, U.S. Army War College, 2004. http://www.dtic.mil/cgi-bin/GetTRDoc?Location=U2&doc=GetTRDoc.pdf&AD= ADA424088 (accessed 27 October 2010).

Donegan, S., R. Bellamy, and C. L. Gamble. ―Vaccines for Preventing Anthrax.‖ Cochrane Database of Systematic Reviews 2009, Issue 2. Art. No: CD006403. DOI: 10.1002/14651858.CD006403.pub2. http://www2.cochrane.org/reviews/ en/ab006403.html (accessed 20 March 2011).

Emergent BioSolutions. ―BioThrax® (Anthrax Vaccine Adsorbed).‖ http://www.fda.gov/ downloads/BiologicsBloodVaccines/BloodBloodProducts/ApprovedProducts/Lic ensedProductsBLAs/UCM074923.pdf (accessed 2 September 2010).

———. ―Emergent BioSolutions Awarded HHS Contract Valued at up to $186.6 Million to develop rPA Anthrax Vaccine.‖ http://investors.emergentbiosolutions.com/ phoenix.zhtml?c=202582&p=irol-newsArticle&ID=1472596&highlight= (accessed 11 February 2011).

Federal Bureau of Investigation. ―Amerithrax Investigation.‖ http://www.fbi.gov/anthrax/ amerithraxlinks.htm (accessed 15 September 2010).

McMichael, William H. ―Review Ordered for Anthrax Vaccine Refusers.‖ *Army Times*, 26 April 2008. http://www.armytimes.com/news/2008/04/SATURDAY military_anthraxvaccines_042608w/ (accessed 12 November 2010).

Melik, James, and Anbarasan Ethirajan. ―Anthrax Outbreak Hits Bangladesh Leather and Meat Sectors.‖ *BBC News*, 13 October 2010. http://www.bbc.co.uk/news/ business-11451570 (accessed 17 October 2010).

Nass, Meryl. ―Surveillance Program for Short-Term Health Effects of AVA.‖ http://www.anthraxvaccine.org/NassDOD.htm (accessed 12 November 2010).

Penslar, Robin L. "Office for Human Research Protections (OHRP) IRB Guidebook." U.S. Department of Health and Human Services. http://www.hhs.gov/ohrp/ irb/irb_guidebook.htm (accessed 30 September 2010).

Rempfer, Thomas L. "Anthrax Vaccine as a Component of the Strategic National Stockpile: A Dilemma for Homeland Security." Master's thesis, Naval Postgraduate School, Monterey, California, 2009. https://www.hsdl.org/homesec/ docs/theses/09Dec_Rempfer.pdf (accessed 12 November 2010).

Roos, Robert. "FDA Seeks Comments on Controversial Anthrax Vaccine." Center for Infectious Disease Research and Policy Academic Health Center, University of Minnesota. http://www.cidrap.umn.edu/cidrap/content/bt/anthrax/news/ jan1305anthrax.html (accessed 11 November 2010).

Vaccine Healthcare Centers Network. "About the Vaccine Healthcare Centers Network (VHC)." http://www.vhcinfo.org/aboutUs.asp?page=about&title=About Us&subnav=about (accessed 3 January 2011).

www.ingramcontent.com/pod-product-compliance
Lightning Source LLC
Chambersburg PA
CBHW081207180526
45170CB00006B/2246